HEAL

A Psychiatrist's Inspiring Story of What it Takes
to Recover from Chronic Pain, Depression, and
Addiction...And What Stands in the Way

BY SUMTER M CARMICHAEL MD

ISBN: 1479230405
ISBN-13: 9781479230402
Library of Congress Control Number: 2012916437
CreateSpace Independent Publishing Platform
North Charleston, South Carolina

The events that follow actually happened, but the names and details of the stories have been altered to protect the privacy of the individuals.

TABLE OF CONTENTS

Acknowledgments   ix

Foreword by Dr. Nancy Qualls-Corbett   xiii

Introduction   1

PATIENTS ARE THE BEST TEACHERS

Chapter One: Learning From Patients   7
   What Patients Face When They Try to Get Help with Pain

Chapter Two: Encounters with Pain and Addiction   17
   Learning from Addicts: The Importance of the Doctor-Patient
   Relationship

Chapter Three: Discovering How Pain Works   23
   Lessons from Teaching Pharmacology

ENCOUNTERS WITH MEDICINE GET PERSONAL

Chapter Four: I Get Multiple Sclerosis   33
   I Discover What Living with MS and Depression Really
   Means

Chapter Five: The Wounded Healer: Lessons Learned   41
   After an Injury, I Get Chronic Pain and Struggle to Get Well

EMOTION: THE KEY TO UNDERSTANDING

Chapter Six: Expanding My Understanding of How Medicine Works   57
    An MS Clinic Teaches Me the Importance of Emotion and
    I Learn the Health Benefits of Food

Chapter Seven: The Story of Inborn Anxiousness and Pain   63
    How Migraines, Mitral Valve Prolapse, Temporomandibular
    Joint (TMJ), Irritable Bowel Syndrome (IBS), and
    Fibromyalgia Fit Together

Chapter Eight: Physical Problems Get Confused with
                 Unconscious Responses to Anxiety   75
    Sorting out Manifestations of Anxiety from Physical
    Illness

Chapter Nine: Unravelling the Mystery of Anxiety   83
    Anxiety and All the Creative Ways Anxiety Shows Itself in
    the World

Chapter Ten: Cultural Illusions   89
    Understanding How Beliefs Help Us or Get in Our Way

Chapter Eleven: Placebos and Nocebos   93
    Understanding the Doctor's Role in Healing

FINDING THE PATH TO RECOVERY

Chapter Twelve: Lessons from the Poor and from Young Doctors   107
    I See Medical Patients with Depression and Teach Medical
    Students

Chapter Thirteen: Finding the Path to Recovery   117
    Finding What Works Even When Resources are Limited

Chapter Fourteen: The Depression-Pain Connection   125
    Understanding How Pain and Depression Go
Hand in Hand

Chapter Fifteen: Starting a Program for Pain and Depression   133
    Patients Respond to Simple Interventions

Chapter Sixteen: The Unfolding Addiction Problem   141
    Many with Pain and Depression Have Addiction Issues

Chapter Seventeen: Preparing for the New Endorphin Clinic: 147
    Understanding Addiction, Tolerance and How
Best to Use Opiates

Chapter Eighteen: Harm Reduction: The Treatment
                  Program for Addicts   157
Developing a Program for Addicts with Pain and
Serious Illness

Chapter Nineteen: The Endorphin Clinic Treatment Program   163
    Making the Treatment of Pain Effective, Patient
Friendly and Affordable

Chapter Twenty: Emotional, Social and Occupational
                  Rehabilitation   173
Understanding the Road to Recovery

Chapter Twenty-One: Spiritual Rehabilitation   179
    The Key to Recovery from Chronic Pain,
Depression, and Addiction

Chapter Twenty-Two: The Fifth Vital Sign   185
    Where Medicine Went Wrong

PHYSICIANS, HEAL THYSELVES!

Chapter Twenty-Three: Doctors Are Not Getting the Word   191
    How Psychiatry Failed to Listen to Itself

Chapter Twenty-Four: The Doctor's Influence on
                       Self-Defeating Behavior   199
    Can Empathy Be Taught?

FINAL THOUGHTS

Chapter Twenty-Five: And They Lived Happily Ever After   211
    Finding New Life after Loss: Love, Joy, and Creativity

Appendix A: Unconscious Defense Mechanisms: 215
Appendix B Medical Conditions That Give Rise to Depression   221
Appendix C Medications That May Cause Depression   223
Appendix D Symptoms of Depression   225
Appendix E Plan for Treating Bad Pain Periods   227

ACKNOWLEDGMENTS

My debt of gratitude stretches from childhood through my own struggles with multiple sclerosis (MS) and chronic pain, my experience putting together a pain clinic for the poor, and my struggles with writing this book. To my mother and grandmother, I owe thanks for their courageous model in dealing with life's most difficult challenges. I am thankful to my mentors in medicine and psychiatry, especially Dr. A. H. Russakoff and Dr. Clark Case, who taught me soulful lessons about being a doctor. These physicians always recognized the individuality of the persons they were treating and understood the effect of that personhood on illness and pain. And I thank the generations of medical students and young doctors, interns, and medical residents whose questions challenged my thinking. I am also grateful to the internists and neurologists who sent me patients—and especially for their willingness to learn about the way the emotions and the body interact.

A special thanks is due to Dr. Max Michael, who encouraged me to come to the county hospital and teach medical students and young doctors about pain, anxiety, and depression. My thanks to Dr. Sandral Hullett and the medical staff at Cooper Green Hospital, who allowed me to organize and operate a multidisciplinary pain clinic program for the poor and uninsured. And thanks to the staff and patients who assisted me in making that possible. A special thanks to Jane Trechsel, who not only expanded my worldview and shared her special knowledge with me and my patients, but allowed me to hone and polish my words with her insightful comments. Thanks to the many volunteers who contributed their special skills to teaching patients and staff a better way to eat, move, meditate, and be. Many thanks to Dan Doleys, PhD; Nancy Qualls-Corbett, PhD; and Anne Xavier, MD, who shared their wisdom with me.

As for the manuscript, I am greatly indebted to my husband, Steve Coleman, for his help and encouragement in making the words take shape. Without his help, I would not have a book. A special thanks to friends and colleagues who read the book and gave me feedback and ideas, especially Marjorie White, who made a detailed review; Lyn Stafford, who pulled the book together when I was lagging, and Wodie Monaghan and Anne Miller, who made insightful comments, and Deborah Young and Judy Prince who reviewed my final document.

Thanks, to all who taught me, inspired me, and encouraged me along the way. I have benefitted from the wisdom of many, but none wiser than the patients who shared their lives and struggles with me. They were my ultimate teachers of compassion, humility, and the need to listen, thus helping me to understand the complexities of chronic pain: what it takes to recover and what stands in the way.

To all those patients over the years who have inspired me to write this book, and to my grandchildren, Colin and Ian, Eva and Annie. Here are pearls from my heart.

FOREWORD

"Existence is suffering," proclaims the first noble truth in classical Buddhist meditations. As difficult as these words are to acknowledge, we recognize that life is not without various degrees of suffering and pain. Pain is an integral aspect of all human existence. Pain is experienced in all cultures and by all creeds and colors of humankind. It is universal. As much as we choose to deny it or to hide from it, pain is our common heritage. When confronting physical or emotional pain, our outlook on life is diminished, our personality is altered, and our relationship with others deteriorates. Pain can control our very being as we despairingly succumb to that which seems beyond our physical or emotional control.

From legend and lore, we know that pain has existed since the beginning of time; we also find that treatments for the alleviation of pain are age-old. Ancient civilizations knew this principle well. The ancient Greeks left us the mythological wounded healer, Chiron. He was a majestic centaur, half man and half horse. The epitome of strength, this beautiful creature was the paradigm of one who is in touch with the invaluable instincts of animal nature while at the same time attuned to the human intellect and healing knowledge. Chiron was known as the wounded healer because he was unable to heal his own trauma. Yet through his grief and anguish, he was able to recognize and empathize with the pain in others in order that they might be cured. He taught the healing arts to Asclepius and Heraclitus. These wise ancient figures foreshadow the healers of modern times.

In Epidaurus, Greece, we find the ruins of the Temple of Asclepius, the Greek god of healing. There, we see small cubicles where those who suffered physical and emotional pain were attended to by the priests of Asclepius and were healed in body and soul.

The Greek healer Hippocrates, known as the father of medicine, gave us the art of caring for psyche and soma and an appreciation of the tremendous battle one endures when debilitating pain inflicts one's personhood. Fortunately, medical science and the modern-day "priests of Asclepius," our physicians and health care therapists, have made numerous advances in alleviating pain. Miracle drugs and therapeutic remedies have brought blessed relief to our numerous painful afflictions. But there is more than just a quick remedy needed to heal our pain.

A wounded healer herself, Dr. Sumter Carmichael has explored in this book the many pathways, from physical to spiritual, approaching the complex issue of pain. Through her knowledge, experience, and heartfelt wisdom, she is a guide offering a gentle yet resourceful light into the dark abyss of pain.

Dr. Nancy Qualls-Corbett

INTRODUCTION

The body has the wisdom to heal, but it requires of us reengagement in life: exercise, work, and love.
—Sumter M. Carmichael, MD

A vast industry now exists to help us cope with pain. Since 1999, great effort has been exerted to identify patients who are suffering unnecessarily. Doctors have been asking everyone to rate their pain level from one to ten on every visit to the doctor. Every community has pain clinics approaching pain from every possible angle. There are books, blogs and specialty magazines on every topic related to pain. Still, too many suffering individuals fail to get the help they need to recover from pain, depression, and the debilitating effects of chronic illness, while too many doctors pursue a course that threatens the first principle on which medicine rests: *do no harm.*

Real Pain

In medical school, and then residency in psychiatry, I observed the difficulty doctors had dealing with emotion and seeing patients as human beings struggling with human problems. Dazzled by astonishing scientific and technological advances, doctors embraced the illusion that they can solve the problem of human illness with sophisticated medical testing combined with pills, shots and surgery. Ambiguous problems or those not fitting into this approach present a particular problem for doctors, even psychiatrists. It seemed to me, even early on, that a failure to understand the important role of emotion in our lives and illnesses was the basis for this difficulty, but that was not completely clear to me then.

I began medical school in 1960. The McCarthy witch hunts were just past. The war in Vietnam was underway and the civil rights protests were beginning. The women's liberation movement was still a decade away. In those days there was much debate about which conditions had a physical basis and which had a psychological one, the latter clearly of lesser import if not a nuisance altogether. If doctors thought a patient had a psychological problem rather than a physical one, they might belittle that patient and dismiss the complaint instead of investigating the psychological symptom as they would any physical symptom *to find its underlying cause.* This tendency to ignore how emotion was affecting the patient and the illness was especially acute if the patient's physical condition was hard to pin down as it so often is when pain is involved.

I first encountered this prejudice against emotion and the potential for devastating results at age sixteen when I developed recurrent bouts of stomach pain from appendicitis. The doctor thought it was just *nerves* and told me to drink prune juice every day. On return visits every three or four weeks he would laugh at my being out of school again. This continued until one night I had a shaking chill and my mother recognized her own symptoms with appendicitis and took me to have my appendix out. By failing to explore the basis of the nervous symptom he thought I had, my doctor had missed a diagnosis that cost my paternal grandmother her life in 1906. And by laughing at me instead investigating the source of my nervous complaint, he missed an opportunity to give me tools to deal with whatever was troubling me. He certainly taught me that when dealing with the medical profession, it is better to have what doctors call *real disease:* something that can be measured, seen with the eye or held in the hand!

Today we have come a long way in understanding how the brain works. We even know that emotion is essential to making decisions. Even so, doctors still fight the physical-versus-psychological battle when it comes to conditions that cannot be measured by a test, especially chronic illnesses that include symptoms of pain and depression. The problem is aggravated by changes in the medical system. Over the past twenty-five years, I have watched as doctors have become more anxious about malpractice suits and the loss of income from third party payers, especially

Medicare. As a result doctors have begun focusing on ways to manage risk in their practices and maximize profit by hiring ancillary personnel to handle many tasks. That means doctors spend less time with patients, and rely more on expensive tests to detect serious conditions. It also means that interpretations of a patient's behavior and symptoms are more easily distorted by the doctor's own prejudices and unconscious responses to anxiety. Many complaints that take a patient to the doctor go unaddressed or overmedicated. This has devastating effects on the cost and practice of medicine today and has even crept into the practice of psychiatry, which has sought more and more to fashion itself after medicine.

In this climate, pressures on physicians to be more aggressive in their management of pain has spawned an explosion in opiate prescriptions, even when other interventions would be better for the patient. In response to the demand, pharmaceutical companies have produced ever more potent opiates. Addiction is rampant. Most opiates are being supplied by pain clinics and prescriptions from primary care physicians, internists, and dentists. The death rate from opiate overdoses in this country now rivals the deaths from car accidents in many states.[1] Since I started writing this book, the use of medication for pain has skyrocketed. The United States has 4.6% of the world's population and as of 2012, Americans consumed 80% of all the world's opioids, and 99% of the hydrocodone.

This book, which chronicles what I discovered in the course of my medical career and life with multiple sclerosis, chronic pain and depression, sheds light on what is needed to recover from illnesses where pain, anxiety, depression, and self-defeating behaviors such as inactivity, overeating, smoking or other addictions dominate the picture. It explores the difficulty physicians have when faced with pain and other conditions where no measure exists except the subjective one. This book discloses the underlying factors involved in the over reliance on technology in the practice of medicine today. And it explores the reasons for the resistance to age-old, culturally-tested healing remedies. This is my lifetime of

---

[1] Karen Hanson, "A Pill Problem: Prescription Drug Abuse is the Fastest Growing Form of Substance Abuse" State Legislatures 36.3 (2010) 22–24. Expanded Academic ASAP.Web. 20 Sept. 2010.

discovery of what is involved in the healing process and what has gone wrong in modern day America.

I am writing this book for the general public, especially those with chronic pain or depression who feel stuck. They may have tried everything and just are not getting better. I am writing for those who do not understand what pain, and especially chronic pain, is all about and what the role of the medical profession needs to be to get them better. I am explaining what is involved in the recovery process from any chronic illness, especially where pain, depression and addictionn are involved. And I am writing to all those people who still think that physical pains are real and emotional ones are not. I am writing to all those people who do not understand how emotions work, what the placebo effect really amounts to, and why opiates are a blessing and a curse. And I am writing to those who still think addiction is a plague brought on us by sinners and the poor.

In addition, I am writing for doctors and would-be doctors. I hope to show them how to understand emotion, both positive and negative emotion, including pain, and how to use that knowledge to further healing without taking a lot of time. I want to alert them to the cultural battle being fought in the guise of standard medical practice and I want to wake them up to the big mistakes being made in the treatment of chronic pain and depression today.

I would like to say to doctors, "Forget the medical model and listen hard to what the patient is saying, what the patient wants!" Doctors and patients sometimes forget that it is anxiety that takes the patient to the doctor—not bleeding, fever, or pain! And addressing the patient's concerns may be not only most efficacious for that patient, but cost effective to boot. Doctors too often forget that healing comes from within, and that the doctor's influence on that inner healing process involves more than making diagnoses and giving pills.

My second book, *Heal Thyself: What You Can Do to Recover from Chronic Pain and Depression*, contains a practical guide that covers in detail what patients can do to assist their doctors to manage their own pain and depression. Both doctors and patients with chronic illnesses will find it useful. Pain and suffering, and all that surrounds them, are subjects that touch us all.

PATIENTS
ARE
THE
BEST
TEACHERS

CHAPTER ONE

LEARNING FROM PATIENTS

The most essential part of a student's instruction is obtained not in the lecture room, but at the bedside. Nothing seen there is lost; the rhythms of disease are learned by frequent repetition; its unforeseen occurrences stamp themselves indelibly in the memory.
—Oliver Wendell Holmes, MD

I took my medical training at Cornell's impressive New York Hospital with rotations at Bellevue hospital on the East River in New York City. One could not help but be in awe at the impressive medical structures and the armies of white-clad men who addressed life's most serious concerns. I was certainly impressed and tried to look very professional behind my little white coat, though as I was one of a few women students I could not help but stand out. The head of surgery had told me I didn't belong there, though that may have been because I was doing too well on the surgery rotation. I suppose even to me, I was just in medicine because my *real* life of marriage and children had yet to begin. Still medicine was fascinating. As an outsider, for I certainly didn't feel like *one of the boys*, it felt like visiting an era from the past or a foreign country for the first time. Even my mother called the first day to alert me that there were *men living in the building.* It was a man's dorm. The women had the second floor. It was a man's world and I felt privileged to walk the same halls where generations of physicians had been trained. The lecture halls were from the nineteenth century and Victorian aged Bellevue still had thirty-five bed wards.

This was a heady time in the medical profession with a great feeling of optimism. Dr Jonas Salk found a vaccine to cure polio, and the sense was that medical science was on track to cure all disease. Still in every room were patients facing challenging issues: children with cancer, unmarried women having babies at a time when that was considered shameful, and many dying from heart disease, bleeding ulcers, and Lou Gherig's disease. In addition cancer surgery was extreme: such as, hemi-pelvectomies for bone cancer with seeming little concern about how the patient would feel about life after that radical surgery.

Being an outsider, as I certainly was, freed me to see some problems along the way. I could not help but notice the impersonal way patients were treated on rounds. Any expression of emotion was seen as lack of cooperation or *female hysteria* by the attending physicians. I began making mental notes. Even after my transfer to Alabama for a medical internship year with Dr. Tinsley Harrison on my way to Boston for my residency in psychiatry at the distinguished Massachusetts General Hospital, I observed the impersonal way patients were treated. When I married later that year, we stayed in Alabama, my husband's home, rather than move to Boston, and I eventually took my residency in psychiatry there.

The medical world's insensitivity and difficulty with emotion was again brought home to me one day during my training in psychiatry when I was asked to see a patient in the Comprehensive Cancer Center at the University of Alabama in Birmingham (UAB) who appeared to be demanding pain medicine she should not have needed. The patient, Mrs. Emily Griffin, was lying in her hospital bed, glaring at a blank television, when I got to her room. Her roommate was retching in the bathroom, and the noise and smells were disconcerting. I pulled the curtain to get some privacy, wishing there was another place we could talk.

"She's having chemotherapy," Mrs. Griffin began, nodding toward the bathroom. She looked back at me and listened to my introduction. "Do the doctors think I'm crazy? Is that why they've sent me a psychiatrist?" I tried to reassure her and focus on her pain. "Is that why they called you?" she went on. "I have breast cancer. Five years ago, they removed my breast. It took me a long time to get over being sick from chemo and come to terms with the changes, but I did, and I've been teaching again for the last two years. I've nearly made it to the five-year mark." She looked away, remembering her anticipation of that important milestone. "Two months ago, I started to hurt." She indicated her chest near her surgery. "The doctors say it may be nothing, so I decided to wait until the end of the term to come in for tests. If the tumor is back, I'll have to have chemo again." Her voice was steady, but I could see the fear behind her reasonable-sounding words. She said she had been teaching every day and taking no pills for pain. "I didn't even want them until I came here for more tests." She shifted position in the bed.

"I don't understand why, when I ask the doctor for something for pain, he won't give me what I want. I had a narcotic for the pain when I was here before, with some Valium for my nerves. That made a huge difference. I don't see why they won't give me what I know will help. When I ring, the nurses take an hour to get here, and then it's just aspirin, which does nothing."

It turned out that the doctor had given Mrs. Griffin aspirin because she had not complained of pain before coming to the hospital. Now, as she became more and more demanding of something stronger, her doctors became convinced that this was inappropriate behavior and refused her requests. The patient's demands made the nurses nervous. They talked about her behind her back. They refused to be manipulated by her demands.

I can still hear the medical resident asking, "How is it that she's been doing fine at home without any medicine? Now all of a sudden, she needs something for pain—and something strong?"

"That's a good question," I replied. "The answer lies in *understanding the patient's experience.* Here she is, anxiously awaiting the results of her tests, away from her routine activities that distract her from worries and pain. She is no longer surrounded by familiar people who help her bridge the uncertainties in her life. Instead, she's effectively imprisoned in a strange place, exposed to patients who are sick and dying, and being ministered to by a staff of people she doesn't know and who don't trust her enough to give her the kind of medicine that helped her before. The whole experience is alienating. Is it any wonder that she's scared and hurting more?"

When I explained the situation in this manner to her physicians and nurses and assured them that she had no history of addiction or drug abuse, they relaxed and gave her opiates for pain relief and Valium for her nerves and to help her sleep. Even though her cancer had come back, after she went home, her pain immediately became manageable again without the use of opiates. Apparently while she was in the hospital, uncertainty about the future made her anxious, and with nothing to distract her, she had more pain. Once at home, she was able to plan her routine and focus on other things, which lessened her pain and her anxiety.

Today, most oncologists recognize *pseudo-addiction*—that is when demanding behavior represents pain that is inadequately treated, not addiction. They also understand that fear, anxiety, and depression not only can make pain worse, but can also give rise to pain on their own.

Nonetheless, patients who are angry often provoke the medical staff, who may themselves get angry and cease to maintain a professional attitude—that is, to remain focused on what is going on with the *patient*. Ron Bowen, a forty-two year old married man, was admitted to the hospital after he tried to kill himself by taking an overdose of insulin. When I first went to see him, Ron was sullen, and angry that his life had been saved.

"I don't understand why I wasn't just left alone to die. I've had diabetes all my life, it seems," he said, looking down where his legs had once been. "I lost my legs ten years ago. I guess I didn't take care of my diabetes well enough when I was young." He moved his position and looked out of the window. "I've had trouble working since then because I hurt so much. Still, my wife stuck it out, but two weeks ago she told me she'd had enough. I've pleaded with her, but she says she's going to move back to Kentucky. I'm tired of trying to make my life work. I hurt in the stumps, and I keep feeling my whole leg is burning even though it's not there anymore."

As we talked, Ron relaxed and a winsome smile appeared on his face from time to time. He and his wife had had a good life together. Both liked country music, and Ron was a bit of a comic. "We used to go out all the time, but recently I hurt so much I've haven't been inter-ested. And I get pissed off easily." As Ron stared out the window at the gathering dusk, I could see how far pain and depression had derailed his life. After we talked some more, I described what we had to offer him. I told him I would leave the care of his diabetes and his leg pains to the diabetes doctors.

Two days later, I was sitting in my office in the outpatient clinic. My secretary came in looking scared. "One of your patients from the hospital is out here threatening to kill himself if you don't see him right away. Shall I call security to take him back to the hospital?"

"You'd better bring him in," I responded, knowing that whoever it was needed my attention right away. When I saw Ron, it was easy to see he was not suicidal. He was just angry and frustrated, not knowing where to turn for help.

"Those stupid diabetes doctors refused to give me any pain medi-cine," he blurted out. "I didn't know what to do." He sat in the chair I indicated across from me and continued his tirade. "I told them I wouldn't take any diabetes medication if they didn't treat my pain. And all the doctor said was, 'Well, if you won't take your insulin, I won't treat you,' and stormed out of the room. So what do I do now? I have to find someone to help me."

I knew that as this man's primary doctor, it was my responsibility to try to find the answer. Yes, I would have to help Ron find better ways of dealing with frustration than taking a hand full of pills or threatening to kill himself, but for the moment, he needed someone to believe in him…and relief from pain.

"I don't know how to treat the pain in your legs," I told him. "That's not my field. But I'll give you a shot of pain medicine now so you can get some relief. Then I'll find out who can help you with a long-term plan." I called the hospital nurse to give him a shot of the opiate Demerol (Meperidine) as soon as he got to the ward.

Even as I did this, I was worried that he might use suicide threats to persuade me to give him more opiates. On the surface, I was taking him at face value, but inside I was affected by the same doubts that had troubled his diabetes doctor. To my surprise, Ron did not ask me for any more pain medication. It took me several days to find someone to help him, and every day I was afraid he would be angry again or want another shot, but he seemed content and asked me for nothing. Finally I found a physician who agreed to work with Ron. He connected Ron to a transdermal stimulation (TENS) unit. Later, Ron told me gratefully that this had given him relief from his pain for the first time in ten years. Ten years!

As a result of my training, I had known to listen to Ron and not just react impulsively or angrily to his inappropriate threats or behavior, even though my doubts were just as strong as those of his other doctors. It was not until I saw his face—the relief and gratitude he had for the help—that I knew how fortunate I was that I had not given in to my own anxiety. What would have happened if I had reacted another way? What if I had called security to fetch this suicidal man who had left the hospital against medical advice? What if I had put him in seclusion—or worse, in restraints? I might even have upped his current medication. Those would have been fairly standard responses, but they would all have been responses to my own anxiety—and therefore less than helpful to this patient.

This encounter taught me the importance of having faith in the patient, even when his or her behavior seems excessive—even when the patient may be looking for drugs. It is not a question of not being fooled. Doctors need to see through lies, but trust is essential to the doctor-patient relationship. It may even be the *one indispensable ingredient in helping patients do better.*

The other thing I found was that doctors are as apt to be anxious and to overreact to stressful situations as their patients. This means doctors are as likely to react out of their own biases and prejudices in these situations as their hapless patients. Angry and demanding people are difficult for anyone, but angry patients may be afraid or depressed. It makes no sense for the doctor, or anyone, to argue or try to reason with them. It is better to listen and *respond to the inner fears they express with their anger.*

I also know that a few doses of an opiate are not going to make someone into an addict, so I can trust what the patient is telling me. Seeing the importance of listening to the patient's point of view reinforced in this way was a good lesson for me as a young physician. It helped me develop a better sense of empathy with patients and taught me not to react to my first fears. Still, I had a long way to go to understand emotion and all the factors involved in the treatment of chronic pain.

The Magic of the Doctor-Patient Relationship

The best example I saw of how the interplay between a patient's anxiety symptoms and a doctor's own anxiety could ratchet up defensive responses was when I was on call one weekend. Mrs. Wilma Berry, who had heart disease, was admitted for three-vessel bypass surgery. While recovering, she became depressed and was transferred to the psychiatric unit to keep her from hurting herself. She had been given a tricyclic antidepressant (TCA) by her psychiatrist, Dr. Linton. This medicine contributed to a drop in blood pressure when she stood up. For that reason, she was ordered to stay in bed. She also had difficulty urinating—another side effect of tricyclic antidepressants. Periodically, she had to be catheterized. Additionally, she had periodic chest pains, which had prompted her cardiologist to leave instructions for an electrocardiogram (EKG) to be taken whenever the pains occurred.

My first introduction to Mrs. Berry came early in the morning. The staff told me she had gotten up from her bed, fallen, and hit the back of her head. She already had been sent for an X-ray, which showed no fracture. After reviewing her chart, I went to see her. Mrs. Berry was sitting up straight in the bed, yelling at the nurses who were trying to put restraints on her arms.

"If you hadn't taken so long to get in here with the bedpan, I wouldn't have tried to get up," she fussed at the nurses. "I don't need to be tied down. I'm not an idiot, but I don't want to wet the bed either." She glared at me. "What do you want? I suppose they think I'm crazy and need to see a psychiatrist. What a bunch of idiots you all are."

"I came to see if you were all right," I answered, examining her head.

"My head is fine. It's these incompetent people up here that are driving me crazy. Tying me down now? What else do I have to endure?"

Mrs. Berry was clearly very conscious and alert. I convinced the nurses that she did not need restraints, admonished her to stay in her bed, and dashed back to my other duties in the emergency room.

Several hours later, I was called to see Mrs. Berry again. This time, she was having chest pain. As I walked in, Mrs. Berry was lying flat in the bed, connected to the EKG machine by multiple wires. "What do you think you're doing?" she complained to the nurse taking the tracing. "It took you all so long to get in here, the pain has already stopped. What kind of a show are you running in this place?"

Hearing her say the pain was gone, I focused on her EKG tracing. Finding it unchanged, I dismissed Mrs. Berry from my mind and returned to the emergency room to see another patient.

A third call about Mrs. Berry came in at nine o'clock that night. She was complaining of pain in her abdomen; she couldn't void. I thought about having her catheterized as the attending physicians had done, but because I didn't want to be part of her litany of complaints the next day, I thought I had better see her first.

The instant I walked in, Mrs. Berry started her tirade about the nurses, doctors, and everything in the hospital. "I don't see how you expect anyone to get well in this place. They test you and stick you, and no one even speaks. Wake you up at all times, but want you to stay in bed and not move about. The nurses are incompetent, and the doctors aren't much better." She droned on, not even looking at me.

I thought, *Why didn't I just catheterize her? That's what all the other doctors did when she couldn't void. She has medicine side effects. I know depressed people are difficult and testy, but this is just too much. She's so unpleasant; no wonder no one wants to have anything to do with her.* I was sorely tempted to simply get up and leave. But remembering the voice of my mentor in psychiatry, *"Stay focused on the patient and what the patient's behavior says about her,"* I struggled to say something empathetic instead. *There must be something that can shift the focus off her harangue,* I thought as I watched her.

"How have you stood all of that?" I asked, finally.

Mrs. Berry looked at me for the first time and began to tell me about her life. "My husband divorced me twenty years ago to marry a younger woman and moved to Oregon. My boys were teenagers then and went to live with him. He had all the money. He should have had to give me something, but he hid all his assets. That was all right as long as I could work. I worked in Mobile. My whole family lives there. I was the mayor's executive secretary. I loved it. Loved Alabama politics. Now I can't do that anymore because of my heart. My family has to support me. I know they resent it, and I don't like it much better. This surgery is my last chance for any life at all. But how can I have a life when I can't even get out of bed?" Suddenly, she stopped and looked at me hard. "Do you have a pill for me?" she asked.

I was so surprised by this sudden shift that I could barely speak. She had hit on the problem. After a moment of silence, I spoke. "You know as well as I do that we don't have a pill for being old and sick and useless!" (How many times I have thought of better ways to say that—more precise, more tactful, more sympathetic?)

But her response to my honesty was stunning. I could see her relief that she had finally found someone who understood and did not just dismiss her as a collection of symptoms, either physical or emotional. To my amazement, she was instantly transformed. She actually grinned. We talked for some time, and I found her to be an interesting and delightful woman.

Before leaving the hospital the next morning, I went back to see her. She was still smiling. "I've already seen my cardiologist this morning," she related. "He was surprised to see me smiling. He said he had never seen me smile before. I didn't have any more trouble with my bladder, either. I don't understand why, but talking things out with you helped me get a new perspective. I didn't realize how long I'd been angry and held that all in. I called my cousin in Fairhope this morning. She's an early riser. She's the one I grew up with, and I'm going to go live with her when I leave. She's going to have me transferred to a hospital nearer her home so she can visit me, and I'm going to find doctors who listen to me."

The cardiologist might have been surprised at this patient's transformation, but I was no less so. I knew that being understood is magic and that receiving the kindness and understanding of another is transformative. But until that moment, I had not fully realized that *identifying the real source of the problem* gives the patient a chance to resolve his or her own concerns.

Stress causes physical symptoms. Groups of physical symptoms may be labeled as depression or an anxiety disorder, perhaps completely disguising the real situation behind the scenes. Pills have their place in the treatment of depression and anxiety symptoms, especially when the patient is so overwhelmed that she can no longer work things out on her own, but failure to recognize the source of the stress and help the patient come to terms with it cheats the patient of an opportunity to face reality with a supportive other person, and complicates everything.

When Mrs. Berry had to be kept in bed because her medicine caused a drop in her blood pressure, it generated new problems, which the staff failed to recognize. They saw an unruly and unpleasant patient who troubled them with extra tests and complaints. Instead of recognizing the source of Mrs. Berry's difficulty and helping her, the staff became part of her problem by running too many tests and becoming hostile. For patients with heart problems, such a response may actually increase the chance of a heart attack. For other patients, it may mean unnecessary and expensive tests, a difficult time in a hostile environment, and too much medicine for pain, anxiety, and depression. All of this interferes with the patient's ability to accept the new realities in life resulting from injury or illness, and it retards healing from the surgery or the illness as well.

CHAPTER TWO

ENCOUNTERS WITH PAIN AND ADDICTION

*I will lift mine eyes unto pills. Almost everyone takes
them, from the humble aspirin to the multi-coloured,
king-sized three deckers, which put you to sleep,
wake you up, stimulate and soothe you all in one. It
is the age of pills.*
—Malcolm Muggeridge

Seeing Addiction as Self-Defeating Rather Than Immoral Behavior

My medical and psychiatric training gave me a limited introduction to addiction and addicts. In medical school, we studied about opiates and something about the history of addiction in this country. Doctors were so concerned about preventing addiction that they often underutilized opiates in the treatment of chronic pain except terminal cancer. Most substance abuse programs were based on twelve-step programs like Alcoholics Anonymous (AA) and run by recovering alcoholics and addicts, not psychiatrists.

My initiation to addicts and addiction treatment took place in 1976, when I was asked to serve as the medical director of the federally funded drug abuse program at UAB for a year while they searched for a big name to head up the program. As a young staff psychiatrist, I went where I was told and did my homework by reading all I could find on addiction. During the year I served, Marjorie O'Shea, a surgical nurse, was admitted to the in-patient unit for treatment of opiate addiction.

I first saw Marjorie in the hospital after she had been assessed by the other members of the drug treatment team. "I don't need to talk to you," she said, looking at me defiantly. "I've already been interviewed enough."

Over the next two weeks, she was taken off drugs gradually according to the written protocol. She took part in other parts of the program and even became chummy with other members of the treatment team, but she remained sullen and distant with me.

One day she developed sharp stomach pains due to an ectopic pregnancy about to rupture. She was rushed to surgery. On her return, the surgeon sent instructions: "She'll need opiates, since she'll be in a lot of pain."

Under our agreement with the federal government, we could not give Marjorie opiates for anything but detox, but I did not want to undo the progress she had already made by transferring her off the unit. In the end, I decided to let her make the choice.

"Marjorie," I said, "your surgeons have prescribed opiates for your pain, but to give them to you, we have to discharge you from the unit. Now, I don't want you to suffer, but you've come so far with your treatment that I don't want to mess up your recovery either. So you'll have to let me know how much pain you can take." She looked at me long and hard as I was talking; I was not sure which way she would go.

"I'd like to stay and give it a try," she said.

"Let me know if the pain gets to be more than you can bear," I said, glad she was going to stay. To offset the lack of medicine, I arranged for her to have visits from staff and from other patients. In addition, I visited her myself several times during the day and brought her a magazine or piece of candy so I would be giving her something tangible. At times, I could see she was hurting, but she made it through without the opiates.

In the end, Marjorie thanked me for having faith in her. She admitted that she had not wanted to deal with me in the beginning because she did not really want to be in treatment or to stop using drugs. Now that she had seen that she could live without opiates, she was grateful that she might get her life back and head in a better direction.

That experience taught me how doctor support can help patients avoid dangerous or self-defeating behavior in tough times. If the physician reacts negatively and defensively to the patient's nastiness or negativity, however, he or she will only make the patient more resistant and thereby compound the problem.

I knew that the relationship with me had made a difference to Marjorie. New as I was to addiction treatment (and certainly inexperienced at managing pain), I knew it was my faith in this woman and her basic strength that had helped her. Other members of the team who had wanted me to transfer her off the unit and give her opiates did not understand that some things hurt more than pain. Self-respect, being able to hold your head up, is a powerful motivator, but it is important not to face difficult choices alone. We are all weak at times and need support to put up a spirited resistance.

Lessons from Teaching Pharmacology

During that year, I was asked to lecture to UAB medical students in the sophomore pharmacology course on addiction. One of the hospital patients, a chronic heroin addict, jumped at the chance to tell the class how he conned drugs from emergency room doctors. I directed the discussion and added comments while my patient told his story. The students were fascinated and learned an important lesson.

When the pharmacology department asked me to lecture again the next year, I approached the medical society to help me find a speaker. They found a recovering alcoholic to come talk to the group. This man, a physician in his fifties, was doing a courageous thing just by appearing in public to talk about his alcoholism, because in those days the stigma of being a recovering alcoholic was so great. Prior to 1970, the medical profession did not realize that drug and alcohol problems are an occupational hazard for physicians and other health care providers. A rash of physician suicides in Oregon, following the enactment of punitive laws affecting physicians found to be abusing drugs or alcohol, forced the profession to take a deeper look at the problem. That scrutiny resulted in more realistic steps to deal with the roughly 10 percent of physicians in trouble with drugs and alcohol.

In the past, physicians had been able to hide their addictions for years, but by 1973 cocaine use became rampant on the street, and suddenly young physicians and other professionals were getting into difficulty fast and seeking treatment to keep their licenses. Georgia and Mississippi each developed a program aimed at treating doctors and other professionals with drug problems. For several years, I had groups of young physicians in treatment come from Mississippi to talk to the students.

I would start the session with George Carlin singing about drugs in America, from the caffeine in the morning to the aspirin to that drink at night. Then a panel of six physicians would tell their stories. One could hear a pin drop as they told about their drug and alcohol use in college and medical school. Once I had the attention of the class, I would present the facts about alcoholism and addiction. For the next twelve years, the pharmacology department asked me back to do my dog and pony show with the physician-addicts. For a number of those years, it was the only training medical students got in either drug abuse or alcoholism.

Teaching about addiction turned out to be the back door for me to talk about pain and the clinical use of drugs that get abused. The third year the pharmacology department asked me to add that to my annual routine: teaching about the clinical use of opiates in the treatment of pain, tranquilizers in the management of anxiety, sedatives in the management of sleep, and stimulants in the treatment of depression. Little did I know then how central pain would become to me personally, or to my practice of medicine.

Teaching about Pain

Preparing for my lectures in pharmacology each year, I read everything I could find about pain and the causes of pain and addiction.

Medical researchers were still trying to separate the effects of the mind from the reactions of the body like trying to determine how much pain was physical and how much was psychological, or where to draw the line—as if a line could be drawn.

In my teaching I explained to the students that doctors divided pain into two types: acute and chronic. *Acute pains* are those that come on suddenly or gradually and tend to resolve, with or without treatment, in one to three months. They have a variety of causes, that can usually be identified. *Chronic pains*, on the other hand, might be intermittent or steady pains that go on for six months or (for most) much longer. These chronic pains tend to be harder to understand and treat.

I explained that pains were also divided into somatic, visceral, and neuropathic: somatic from the skin, muscles, and tendons; visceral from the organs; and neuropathic from damage to nerves or to the brain. Somatic pains tend to be well localized, either sharp or dull, aching or stabbing. They are treated with non-steroidal anti-inflammatory drugs (NSAIDS) such as aspirin or ibuprofen, steroids, or opiates. Visceral pain, from internal organs, is poorly localized and may be felt in some other part of the body. Heart pain, for example, may appear as cramping in the left arm, neck, or jaw. All these pains that come from sensory nerves are called *nociception.*

Neuropathic pain, on the other hand, I would explain, results from damage to nerves in the body, in the spinal cord, or in the brain itself. Neuropathic pain tends to be burning, tingling, or stabbing, like lightning. It is not well localized to the area of injury. Neuropathic pain is often felt in whichever part of the body is served by a certain part of the nervous system. Phantom-limb pain felt by amputees is of this kind and seems to hurt where the limb is missing. The burning or stabbing pains of diabetic neuropathy are of this kind as well. Neuropathic pain tends to respond best to anxiolytic, antidepressant, or anticonvulsant medications, always with some crossover, of course.

During my years of teaching in pharmacology, researchers discovered the endorphins and the enkephalins, opiate-like substances that occur naturally in our brains. Wow! This was a huge step forward to find our own built-in painkillers! It was clear to me then that the physiological mechanisms even for the psychological aspects of pain and addiction would be unraveled eventually. After all, are we not chemical factories? This was a fascinating time. Science was nipping away at the edges of emotion.

CHAPTER THREE

DISCOVERING HOW PAIN WORKS

To study the phenomenon of disease without books is to sail on uncharted sea, while to study books without patients is not to go to sea at all.
—Sir William Osler

Wisdom from the History of Pain

One year, while preparing for my lecture in pharmacology, I discovered a book about the history of pain treatment by René Fulop-Miller called *Triumph over Pain*.[2] Just like today, early humans had difficulty understanding pain if *the cause was not intuitively obvious.* That left room for theories fueled by anxiety or prejudice, even from the doctors, scientists, philosophers, and religious leaders of the time. Ancient humans may have attributed a deep pain to God's wrath, whereas more modern doctors might have said the patient is is just neurotic or hysterical, but the process is the same: *humans rationalize what they do not understand.* Rationalization makes us feel better that we have an explanation, but it blinds us to the uncertainty in front of us. Most of the time this rationalization is a benign mechanism that allows us to cope with many of life's uncertainties, but when it affects patients adversely, doctors had better take heed.

---

[2] René Fulop-Miller, *Triumph over Pain* (New York: The Literary Guild of America, 1938).

Reading Fulop-Miller, I discovered that treatments for chronic pain have always included religious and spiritual approaches as well as psychological means to lessen pain and suffering, even as the doctors applied poultices, medicines, and surgery to eradicate treatable problems. I saw, too, that even though each age confronted the fallacies of the age before, attitudes toward pain and patients in pain were always *contaminated by the beliefs of the past* and in particular the beliefs of the healer and the patient. These factors affect treatment right up to the present time. The beliefs of the doctor and the patient affect what treatment is meted out, and what treatment is embraced—sometimes with positive results and sometimes with unfortunate ones, as we will see.

Fulop-Miller reminded me that Jesus and the Christian leaders that followed him were powerful healers. It was only after people began believing more in the science than in religion that the churches' power to heal declined. After reading Fulop-Miller, I began to take a greater interest in the role of belief in healing and pain relief. I knew that belief in medication was important to its effectiveness: an important part of the healing ritual. But I knew how skeptical modern day doctors tended to be about belief.

Again from Fulop-Miller, I learned about belief in the power of touching the sick to relieve pain and suffering, and even to bring people back from the brink of death, has a long history dating back to well before the birth of Christ.[3] Healing by touch continued well into the Middle Ages, even though it became less and less prevalent as fewer believed in it.

During the Middle Ages, some of the power to heal was even transferred to relics such as clothes, utensils, and even dried body parts of the saints. A lively trade in all kind of relics ensued. Ashes, bone, teeth, hands, and fingers of saints and martyrs were in great demand. Those who could help people believe could turn everyday objects and actions into remedies for suffering and pain.[4]

---

[3] Fulop-Miller, *Triumph Over Pain, p*

[4] Fulop-Miller, *Triumph Over Pain*, p

Even in modern times, there have been cases of miraculous healing. The healings at Lourdes, in the 1870s were documented by scientists brought in by the church as being more than a cure for hysterical symptoms.[5] Though questioned by many, reputable scientific men of the time, like Charcot, investigated the curcs and found unexplained instances where tumors had shrunk. Charcot became convinced that suggestion had a powerful effect in reversing the progression of disease.

Even modern medicine has observed instances of unexpected healing following the advent of a new drug treatment. One famous case involved a wealthy man dying of cancer. This man persuaded his doctors to give him the newest drug on the market even though his doctors thought it was too late. His tumors shrank, and he was able to return home. When this same man read a report of the new drug's lack of effectiveness, his tumors reappeared. Having seen this man's miraculous response to the original drug, this time his doctor gave him another drug, saying it was reported to be more powerful than the first. The tumor once more shrank. Only when a final report on the original drug failed to show sustained benefits did this man's tumor return and eventually kill him.[6] Still many remain skeptical about the power of belief.[4]

The Power of Belief

In 1982, I went to China as a guest of the Chinese government. There I saw a patient having his lung removed under acupuncture anesthesia. After the surgery, the man stood up and walked away from the operating table. When I asked the surgeons whether they routinely used acupuncture or Western anesthesia, they replied, "Western anesthesia! You can't take a scared patient into surgery and just stick needles into him. He has to be carefully prepared for acupuncture to work. He has to believe he will not hurt."

---

[5] Anne Harrington, *The Cure Within: A History of Mind-Body Medicine* (New York: W. W. Norton, 2008), 109.

[6] Harrington, *The Cure Within*, 31.

Having grown up in the Episcopal church it had always bothered me that God would only save those who believed in Christ. I would ask myself, *What kind of God would discriminate against the poor people of the world who hadn't even heard of Jesus?* Suddenly I realized that God didn't discriminate. He provided for all the peoples of the world different ways to promote healing and relieve pain. Christianity brings healing if one believes in it.

I saw the same principle at work shortly after my return home from China. My twelve-year-old son asked me, "Why does it make the pain go away when you kiss my hurts?"

"Ah, those are your endorphins, son," said his clever mom. His belief in my kiss was a powerful thing. If ever he stopped believing, the power would go away.

Using the Body's Own Capacity for Healing

Modern Americans sometimes forget that for two thousand years or more, other traditions made use of the body's own capacity for healing and relief of pain. Qigong, for example, is an ancient practice from China that is five to seven thousand years old. The ancients understood that through meditation, guided imagery, and prayer, individuals can eliminate pain and change their lives. For this to work, of course, *one must practice meditation, guided imagery, and prayer*. And to practice, one must believe in the power inherent in these age-old traditions. But even in modern-day America, these practices have much to offer those suffering from pain and depression.

The Role of Emotion

Doctors have always had some difficulty understanding the role of emotion in pain and its connection to medication, particularly opiates. Some of the prejudice about emotion goes back to 1619, when Descartes introduced the concept of the separation of the mind (or soul) and the body. His theory supposedly freed scientists for the first time to treat the emotions and the body separately.[7] The body was seen as a machine that could be studied and manipulated, while psychological events were considered to be supernatural, that is, under the province of God and not under human control. Descartes is also credited with advancing the first theory of pain: that the size of the wound determines the amount of pain experienced. Even though this has been disproven, many physicians today still react as if the amount of damage or the size of the wound determines the amount of pain. That may seem intuitive, but that does not make it true.

Opiates and Emotion in the Treatment of Pain

During World War II on Omaha beach, Dr. Henry Knowles Beecher, then a US Army physician, noticed that the soldiers who were conscious but wounded enough to be evacuated from the beach had very little pain and required few opiates.[6] Even when these wounded soldiers were evacuated to a hospital for further care, only about 20 percent complained of pain, regardless of the extent of their wounds. Yet, only slightly wounded soldiers who were going to be patched up and sent back to the front experienced tremendous pain and required high doses of opiates to control the pain.

When Beecher left the army and went into private practice, he noticed that a much larger percentage of his civilian patients had pain after surgery. He concluded that, for the soldiers, their wounds were their ticket away from danger. His civilian patients, however, had other stresses. Surgery and recovery meant loss of a job, loss of income, and other unpleasant life changes. From these observations, Beecher drew two conclusions: first, that emotion and meaning determine the amount of pain that is experienced, and second, that opiates, the strongest medicines used to treat pain, treat the emotional aspects of that pain.

We now know that in a laboratory setting, where there is no threat of permanent damage or loss, *opiates have no more effect on pain than*

---

[7] Henry K. Beecher, MD, Relationship of Significance of Wound to Pain Experienced. Journal of the American Medical Association 161, no. 17 (1956): 1609–1613.

does water. In laboratory experiments, NSAIDs have been shown to help pain tolerance,[8] but opiates have no effect on pain tolerance at all. In a laboratory setting, the test subject knows there is no threat of permanent damage, so no noxious meaning is attached to the pain. This is the scientific basis for saying that opiates only treat the emotional side of pain, or the meaning of pain. These observations led Beecher to reconsider Descartes' premise that the size of an injury determined the amount of pain felt. Still it was not until the end of the twentieth century that medicine officially recognized that pain and emotion are inseparable.

After World War II, Dr. John Bonica initiated the multidisciplinary pain clinic movement to treat those patients who did not respond to standard medical treatment. In 1973, he founded the International Association for the Study of Pain, which officially recognized for the first time that pain is always an emotional experience and that pain may occur without any actual injury. It defined pain as "an unpleasant sensory and emotional experience associated with actual or potential tissue damage or described in terms of such damage."[9] Even today, many physicians trained to think of pain as the beacon leading to tests that make a diagnosis, think of pain as real only when they can observe it on a test or physical exam, and not when the only evidence is patient reporting. What irony then that the new fifth vital sign[10] is always the patient's subjective report.

Understanding the Way Pain Works

For those who want to understand more about how pain works, the subject of pain was explored in depth by Dr. Paul Brand in his book

---

[8] The maximum amount of pain a laboratory subject can tolerate or as the length of time a subject can endure a noxious stimulus

[9] Bradley Galer, MD and Robert Dworkin, PhD, *A Clinical Guide to Neuropathic Pain* (New York: McGraw-Hill, 2000), 24.

[10] The fifth vital sign, a smily face of how one feels, is requested when pulse, temperature, blood pressure, and respiration are measured.

The Gift that Nobody Wants.[11] Working in India, Brand discovered that lepers lose their limbs because of painlessness. He found that they do not take care of injuries and sores because they cannot feel pain or discomfort, so they end up losing fingers, toes, and more. Brand then came to this country, where he discovered that diabetics lose their limbs for the same reason: if we do not hurt, we do not take care of ourselves. He said that he understood why pain had to hurt so much in order to force a change in our behavior, when he saw an experimental subject turn off a device made to alert him when he was about to injure himself, and continue the same harmful activity. He realized that pain tells us where we begin and where the world leaves off. And he realized that it is pain that tells us when we need to do something different to take care of ourselves.

Brand outlined different levels of pain awareness. First is the pain signal that travels up the nerve into the spinal cord. There, it activates reflexes that remove us from danger. The second level is in the dorsal horn of the spinal cord, the so-called *spinal gate.* Here, pain signals may be suppressed or transferred to the brain, based on signals coming in from the periphery through nerve fibers of different sizes. The final level occurs in the higher brain, which evaluates the incoming pain messages together with other current information, stored memories from childhood, previous pain experiences, and other knowledge; then it directs how much pain we experience, based on the need to get help or take action. Pain best left unfelt until later or not needing immediate attention may be suppressed, while pain needed to change behavior now may be felt right away.

Pain is one of the gifts that wakes us up and gets us to do something different, even if it does not appear to be a gift at the time. Pain that signals a life change may hurt more than pain we interpret as benign, and pain that is severe or persistent may overwhelm us or may damage the nervous system and become chronic. Either chronic pain or being

[11] Paul Wilson Brand and Philip Yancey, Pain: The Gift Nobody Wants (New York: Harper Perennial, 1993).

overwhelmed may lead to an alteration in self-image and bring on depression and self-defeating behaviors.[12]

So, one cannot separate the physical from the emotional when dealing with pain—or any serious illness, for that matter—because the brain is not set up that way. Every move we make, every twinge we perceive, is evaluated by our creative brain and reacted to based on what is happening to us, where we are more vulnerable, and what our past experience has taught us works best. Emotions focus our attention so that we take in more information to deal with a crisis. But even with chronic problems, pain and emotion alert us when we may be hurting ourselves by overdoing or not doing enough.

Today we know that the creative, pliable brain is always learning, modifying, and protecting. It can remove us from peril or dissociate us from the danger that threatens to overwhelm us. It can be damaged by unrelenting pain or depression, as we can now demonstrate with various imaging techniques. But the brain is also capable of regaining what has been lost by relearning to function well. This is the basis of physical therapy through retraining muscles and the brain that manages them. It is also true of other rehabilitation activities: *by acting well in all areas of our lives, we allow the brain to learn to function again in all its myriad ways.*

---

[12] The amount of stimulus required to elicit a pain response is called the pain threshold. The amount of pain an individual experiences is called pain perception, while pain modulation refers to processes in the central brain that regulate the transmission of pain.

ENCOUNTERS
WITH
MEDICINE
GET
PERSONAL

CHAPTER FOUR

I GET MULTIPLE SCLEROSIS

*Suffering has been stronger than all other teaching, and
has taught me to understand what your heart used to
be. I have been bent and broken, but—I hope—into a
better shape.*
—Charles Dickens

The Onslaught Begins

It was my thirtieth birthday, and I was pregnant with my first child. When I bent down to get something off the floor, I had an odd sensation. "What does it mean," I asked my husband, then a resident in neurology, "if I get showers of tingles down the inside of the legs when I tip my head forward?"

He looked at me, alarmed. "I hope you don't have that," he groaned. "Having tingles like that is called L'hermitte's sign, and it means you have multiple sclerosis."

"Oh, I don't have that," I cried in dismay, secretly vowing never to bend my chin down again. In fact, I avoided doing so for months. My pregnancy was happy, and I had a healthy baby girl. When I tested my neck again months later, the tingles had gone. *It must have been the pregnancy, not multiple sclerosis!* I thought gleefully, ready to interpret things the way I wanted them. But the stage had been set.

Two years later, I had another child, a robust little boy. One morning, I noticed my left leg was numb. My husband took me to see a neurosurgeon; he ran tests and found no abnormality. Though neither he nor my husband said anything about multiple sclerosis, somehow I knew. Strange how you can be so wise and fool yourself at the same time.

Once the numbness left my left leg (after about four months), I thought everything was OK. But when the symptoms returned two years later, I decided to see a neurologist who was a specialist in multiple sclerosis.

"This looks ominous," he said. "Come back if anything else develops." He did not use the term *multiple sclerosis*, and neither did I, but the possibility hung in the air like a sword. Again, after a few months, the numbness disappeared, and I was fine. I was busy with the children and getting started in psychiatry. I think the numbness came back briefly for a third time, but I elected to ignore it.

Two years after that, two hours after receiving a flu shot, I lost vision in my right eye. I ran to see an ophthalmologist, who suggested I might have multiple sclerosis. But since the eye got better in a matter of days, and since it was common for that particular flu shot to bring on neurological symptoms, I did nothing further.

It was not until ten years after my first symptom, the week after I took my written psychiatry board examinations, that something truly frightening happened. I was attending a medical meeting in Atlanta. Waiting to step on an escalator, I could not make myself put my foot on the moving steps, no matter how hard I tried. *How odd!* I thought. *I must have an escalator phobia.*

Even so, I went dancing that night in underground Atlanta. Because of the shortage of women at the meeting, I danced every dance and had a wonderful time. The next morning, I woke up with a clumsy left leg, and I could not tell where my foot was in space. *So,* I thought, *It wasn't escalator phobia. It's MS!*

The following day, I went to see another neurologist. This one put me in the hospital to run tests. Computed tomographic (CT) scanning had just become popular, and the neurologist proudly demonstrated the irregularity in my CT scan that confirmed his diagnosis of multiple sclerosis. To me, it looked like a hole in my brain.

While the neurologist looked so pleased at making the diagnosis, he did not seem to notice or care that I was emotionally devastated. He simply announced, "You have multiple sclerosis."

I wanted to scream and cry, but being very controlled, I asked, "What can I do to make the best of this illness?"

Still looking pleased with himself, he turned to me and said, "There is nothing you can do. Cut back on your work; don't burn the candle at both ends. Come back and see me in three months."

Already anxious and depressed, I was already having difficulty concentrating. The abnormality on the CT scan meant to me that I was developing dementia.[13] I was about to lose everything that was of value to me. I did not stop to think about how well I had done on the psychiatry board exams I had just taken or that my difficulty concentrating could be caused by anxiety or depression. No, all I could think was that I was losing brain function. Years later, when another neurologist did an MRI of my brain, I did not have any hole, so I had suffered for nothing. But at the time I learned firsthand of the harm that a doctor's insensitivity can do to a patient. At that moment, getting the diagnosis, but mainly seeing the hole in my head, felt like a death sentence. I was divorced by then, and working part time did not seem possible. Quit my job? And then do what? If I could not support myself, I would not be able to keep my children! The prospect of losing everything I treasured made me feel like my life was over.

I thought back to the first person I had seen with multiple sclerosis during my fellowship at Yale my senior year in medical school. I remembered the horror I had felt watching her sit in a wheelchair in the amphitheater during grand rounds while the doctors talked about her as if she were not there. The other patients presented that morning had all had polio, which was once a scourge, but had since been virtually eradicated by Dr. Salk's vaccine. But multiple sclerosis is still with us. What a heady time that was in medicine, when we thought we could

---

[13] Dementia is the loss of brain function that affects memory and the ability to think. Dementia from multiple sclerosis tends to be a subcortical dementia, which may result in depression or even mania.

eliminate all diseases with vaccines. But that did not happen with multiple sclerosis. Not MS.

If there was nothing anyone could do to treat multiple sclerosis, I could not see the point in coming back to that doctor. He had confirmed what I already knew, and he had added nothing to help me do better. In fact, he had *made me feel worse than was necessary* about my condition. By merely showing me the results of the CT scan without discussing their implications, he failed to explore all my symptoms and created unnecessary worry. From my perspective, doctors who could do nothing useful and only make me feel worse were to be avoided at all costs.

The question of dementia I did take seriously. Immediately, I went to a psychologist to ask about testing how much brainpower I had lost. He laughed and said, "You could lose forty IQ points before it would make any difference." This did not allay my fear that I was losing my mind, but talking about what I was experiencing did help, and I felt confident that he could detect when it was no longer safe for me to practice medicine. I saw him periodically for years.

The Role of Stress

Fortunately for me, not long after this, I attended a lecture at a psychiatric meeting about stress and multiple sclerosis. The doctor who spoke believed that stress made MS symptoms worse, so he advocated many measures to manage stress. In the lecture, I discovered that different stresses can cause pseudo-episodes or worsening of symptoms. It was even possible that the *damage was already there* but only brought to the patient's attention by some stressful event, such as pregnancy, a flu shot, board exams, or a job change. Now I had some hope that I could do something to improve my situation.

Later, I found out that this doctor had been criticized by other specialists in multiple sclerosis because stress had not been scientifically proven to make MS worse. Looking back on more than forty years of experience with the disease, I know that stress of all kinds can bring out my symptoms: the flu, a flu shot, surgery, heat, exercise, overwork, travel, and more. Neurologists call these pseudo-episodes now, since the underlying damage is not actually worse, but to a patient living with the disease, these episodes can be just as difficult and frightening since they affect function.

I Become a Pariah

As soon as my diagnosis of multiple sclerosis was official, I made an appointment to see my boss, the chairman of psychiatry, Dr. Linton. I thought I should tell him I had multiple sclerosis, since I did not know what course would befall me in the future. I did not mention the hole in my head; after all, I had just aced my psychiatric boards. Within a week, I got a letter from Dr. Linton firing me with two weeks' notice! He didn't even know that he could not fire a faculty member on such short notice; I actually had a year to find another job. But since I had been fired, I was removed from my leadership position and my teaching activities. It was difficult trying to work every day, being stuck where I was not wanted. I was already devastated by seeing the hole in my brain, but becoming a sudden pariah did not help.

In retrospect, I can see that I was depressed, but I did not know that then. I could not sleep through the night and had difficulty concentrating, but all I knew was that I felt numb inside. It did not even help to recite to myself what I had accomplished. I still felt like an outcast. Still, I went through my assignments with my head held high. I was to do physical exams in the clinic, so I bought a stethoscope and went off every day to do my new job.

One day, I got a notice about an education meeting. Since I had been in charge of residency teaching the previous year, I took my materials and went. The previous year I had arranged for 167 hours of residency teaching and coordinated that with a psychiatry board training program for all the psychiatrists in the state. Since different people have different learning styles, I had even arranged for activities to appeal to visual learners, auditory learners and experiential leaners. I knew how well the course had been received from feedback I got from lecturers and participants. So I went to the meeting prepared to pass on the information I had amassed. Imagine my shame when Dr. Linton gave out awards to everyone who had even ten hours of teaching responsibility, but did not even mention me or what I had accomplished. He simply announced who was taking over my teaching for the next year. After that, I noticed fewer people saying hello; they either looked another way or crossed the street rather than encounter me.

One day, I confided what I was going through to the man I was dating. I had not told him I had MS before, but felt he cared about me. He seemed supportive when I told him, but over time, I could see that he was calling me less and less. I made excuses for his not calling. Did you think psychiatrists do not fool themselves too? I just went on as if we were still great friends and nothing had really changed. All that ended one day when I walked into a party, and there he was with another woman. After that, I was afraid to tell anyone I had multiple sclerosis. I found myself reading books about stigma. I could still pass as normal, of course; who knows why you limp or may feel down? But I looked differently now at those who were discriminated against. True, I had met discrimination as a woman in medical school, but I did not think that affected my confidence to pursue what I wanted to do or thought was important. Having multiple sclerosis was different. It made me feel vulnerable, and maybe because I was depressed, I did not feel so good about myself anyway.

Finally, after several months, I found a job in the dean's office. The dean set up an office for student programs and made me the affirmative action officer for the School of Medicine. I was charged with representing the interests of the women and minority faculty, staff, and students. I prepared for my job by reading about discrimination in America.

Like most people, I grew up with certain impressions, but had limited knowledge about a lot of issues. Discrimination was one of them. While reading about discrimination, I also read a novel by Leon Uris: *QBVII* is about a German physician who committed atrocities against Jews but also showed great heroism as a doctor in the Far East after the war. Having both German and Southern ancestry, I realized it was *my kind of people* who had been responsible for the misery of so many in this country and abroad. That and my own experience with discrimination made me look differently at those who are the targets of hate.

Ironically, my first assignment as affirmative action officer was to do a study of the School of Medicine for signs of discrimination against women and minorities. The only department showing systematic discrimination against women was the Department of Psychiatry. Years later, the dean asked me why I had not used that information to sue the university for discrimination against me. What I told the dean was that he had treated me well, and that I had felt that it would have been unfair to use information gained as affirmative action officer against the university. I will never forget what he said to me: "You have a shining spirit!" I wrote that down on a small piece of paper to carry with me so I would not forget it. Being depressed as I was for years, it was very hard to feel good about myself, and that small affirmation meant a lot to me.

In the end, the only person I was really able to help during my tenure as affirmative action officer was a woman with Down's Syndrome, who wanted to work but had limited skills and could not compete for a regular job. The government had a special program that allowed the university to pay ten dollars per week for this woman to work in the cafeteria. What a sense of joy she radiated to have a job to go to every day. We forget how much self-esteem for everyone is tied up in being productive and in being able to make a contribution. This knowledge helped me years later when I worked with patients applying for disability who needed to stay disabled to get a government check. Finding a way to be productive, even when one can no longer hold down a full-time or part-time job, is crucial to real recovery from any illness or injury, as well as to having a full old age.

After several years, budget cuts brought an end to my job in the dean's office, and although I returned to the Department of Psychiatry no longer under threat, I knew I needed to move on. In 1980, I went into private practice. Though I was no longer able to teach in psychiatry, I continued teaching in pharmacology, and eventually in the Introduction to Medicine Course in the Department of Medicine.

In medicine my subject was *physician impairment,* a euphemism for drug and alcohol problems, but always my purpose was to give students tools to think. Too often in medicine, doctors act out of their own biases or rote thinking takes over and doctors apply what they know too literally, without considering all the complex factors that affect health and illness. I wanted the young doctors to have a feel for the importance of emotion in being sick or getting well, and I wanted them to understand how cultural beliefs and unconscious responses to anxiety affect our thinking and distort the truth we seek: both in their patients and in themselves. These issues are the core of this book.

During this time, I also initiated a connection between UAB's School of Medicine and the Jefferson County Medical Society's committee on physician impairment. Since I knew that factors other than drugs or alcohol could make it impossible to function as a psychiatrist, I recognized the irony of setting up this working relationship while struggling myself with multiple sclerosis, anxiety, and depression. Still this experience furthered my understanding of addicts and the difficulties they face. Discrimination has a long arm, touching many who have chronic pain, chronic illness, depression, and issues of addiction. If one adds the poor, the uneducated, and minorities, it is a wonder there is anybody left! And that doesn't even count women. Eventually I found a faculty member, himself a recovering alcoholic, to continue the teaching and serve as liaison with the medical society.

CHAPTER FIVE

THE WOUNDED HEALER:
LESSONS LEARNED

Illness is the doctor to whom we pay the most heed;
to kindness, to knowledge, we make promises only; to
pain we obey.
—Marcel Proust

Pain Takes Over My Life

Although I had seen my mother and grandmother deal with pain year after year and had been a physician and psychiatrist for more than two decades, it was not until I endured chronic pain and more depression myself—and tried to find answers in the medical system—that I really began to understand the scope of what patients with pain face and what it takes to recover and fully get one's life back.

One day, fifteen years after my first symptom of multiple sclerosis, I slipped getting out of a canoe and landed hard on my backside. The next day, the pain was so excruciating that I could hardly sit or stand. Even lying down, I hurt if I moved. I contacted the local doctor who had been following my MS. He gave me a shot of cortisone and said he thought I had a slipped disc. He sent me to a neurologist for a myelogram. That test showed no signs of a dislocated disc or any broken bones, so the doctor said he expected the injury would get better with time.

Gradually, I did improve some as I kept working and doing my usual activities, but the pain did not go away, and I had not started jogging again. I knew I was in real trouble that summer when I drove to Cape Cod. I had to stop and walk around every thirty to forty-five minutes because I was in so much pain.

Looking for Answers

When the pain persisted, I went to see my internist for help. He ran a lot of tests that showed nothing wrong. He started me on a regimen of anti-inflammatory medicines for the pain, with little result. The pain made it harder to get around, so I stopped being as active. With less exercise, I started to gain weight. As the pain continued, I went to see an orthopedist, who gave me another shot of cortisone. This helped for a while, but it wore off, and the pain came back.

Although I continued to work as a psychiatrist, I had increasing difficulty walking even to the waiting room to call my patients. I gained more weight and became more depressed. The combination of depression and pain contributed to my withdrawal from activities and friends. At one point I lost interest in nearly everything.

The next time I returned to the orthopedist, he gave me another shot of cortisone and sent me to a physical therapist for a month. The PT applied ultrasound treatments and gave me exercises for my back and leg. The ultrasound actually increased my pain, but the exercises helped a little, and I worked at them diligently. Still, the pain continued, so I went to other doctors looking for relief. I saw a psychiatrist, who gave me talk therapy and medicine for anxiety. Finally, I even went to a rehabilitation doctor to see what I could do to get my life back. That doctor also sent me to physical therapy for a month, where I was prescribed more exercises. By this time, I had gained fifty pounds and felt like the proverbial beached whale.

Next I went to a weight-loss clinic and took off the fifty pounds in six months. I felt better about myself, but still my leg hurt. There was a restless feeling in the muscles that made it hard to sit for long. In addition, a stiff ankle and sharp pains down my spastic leg made walking difficult. Although I managed to go out a little more and had even started dating again, I was limited because I could not sit for long periods without discomfort in my legs. Movies, plays, and concerts were an ordeal or out completely. Even going to work, going on rounds, or sitting in my chair at the office was hard. Being active, going shopping, or enjoying athletic things seemed beyond me.

The Importance of Exercise

Without exercise, the weight started coming back. Now I was desperate. After years of being alone, I was dating; I could not go back to being fat again. I tried everything I could think of to keep the weight off. Somewhere I had read that walking an hour a day would make a difference, so I started to walk up and down the hallway in my home. I thought, *If I'm going to hurt anyway, I might as well walk.* Along the way, I found that when the walking made me hurt more, stretching would lessen the pain for a while so I could go on. I walked, sometimes stopping to stretch every few feet, but I kept going. Gradually, I worked up to walking and stretching for an hour a day, up and down the hall.

After about three months, I decided it was time to transfer my walking to the alley behind my house. The alley is relatively flat and easy to get to. I still remember that first dark morning I set out. The full moon was still high, casting shadows from the giant oak trees to every corner of the garden. It was both beautiful and spooky as I crept up my back steps to the alley. Any fear of walking a dark alley was suddenly allayed when I realized the whole neighborhood was out walking. What a gift to be outside and exercising again! The pain was still there, but I kept moving. Every few feet when I hurt, I would stretch, and I walked the hour.

Once I realized that stretching was essential to reducing my pain, I stretched a lot. When I hurt during the day, I stretched. When I hurt at night, I drank water and stretched some more. Sometimes at night I had to walk off spasms in my weak leg. Drinking a lot of water also helped relieve the spasms. My weight stabilized.

I could tell I was doing better and even asked the neighbors if I could join their morning group walk. I had made it only about ten feet when I was too far behind to continue. It was hard to accept that my desire to join the group was unrealistic, but I did not let that stop me from exercising. I returned to the alley.

Reaching for More

Six months after I had been walking the alley for an hour a day, I met an Ironman. An Ironman is someone who has competed in the Ironman Triathlon. This Ironman was fifty years old and had trained to run twenty-six miles, bike one hundred miles, and swim five miles, all in one day! Awed by his example, I decided to challenge myself to my own version of the Ironman Triathlon. The man I was dating was a long-distance runner, and I wanted to push my limits.

The plan was to add biking and swimming to my walking routine. Biking proved to be too dangerous because of falls, but I did enter a fifty-mile-swim club at a local gym. The gym was across town, so I had to go after work. Although I walked every morning, adding a daily swim to the routine was a challenge. In the beginning, if I swam too much, I was in so much pain that I could not even walk the next day. So to start, I swam every other day and stretched after every length of the pool.

Careful not to overdo, I gradually increased my swim time by no more than 10 percent a week, recording my progress on an activity chart. Measuring the time made more sense for me than trying to keep track of distance. In the pool, I was able to do stretches that I could not manage otherwise. Frequent small stretches seemed to work better for me than big stretches that might make me hurt too much later. The more I stretched, the less I hurt.

Only looking back could I realize how much my pain and spasms were due to tight muscles that needed to be stretched out. For the first time, I could understand treatments like massage therapy and the Feldenkreis Method that stretch the tissues that bind our muscles and add to pain. I learned about stretching for much longer periods of time to be more flexible and how dancers and other athletes may take as much as four hours just to warm up. I realized that most of our efforts to stretch out do not even begin to test what we are capable of doing if we hold stretches for minutes or even hours at a time. Inactivity leads us to hold bent postures for long periods, contributing to shortened muscles and tendons. Depression, desk work, watching television, and other sedentary activities, all lead to the formation of tissue that binds us more and more into stooped positions. Daily stretching and movement are needed just to counteract these trends. To become more flexible, even further effort is required.

As the days passed into weeks then months, the pain in my leg lessened and the restless feeling in my muscles subsided, but if I stopped walking for a day or two, the pain would come back with a vengeance. As long as I exercised and stretched every time I hurt more, I could keep going. As I kept going, my weight stabilized and even decreased.

Spiritual Renewal

Walking and swimming through all the seasons of the year proved to be an amazing experience. Previously, it had been all I could do just to drag myself from my air-conditioned house to my air-conditioned car to my air-conditioned workplace and then back again. I had forgotten the joys of just being outside. I noticed that perspiration evaporated in the hot months to keep me cool and in the cold months formed an additional layer under lots of clothes to keep me warm. I also noticed that after I had been walking for a while, I began to feel like a well-oiled machine.

Still, it was hard to make myself swim every day. The pool was outside, and in winter I had to wear a one-piece ski suit over my wet swimsuit to go from the pool to the gym. Even with a swimming buddy, that was a lonely time because I felt it was so much harder for me than it was for the other athletes. Nevertheless, I did feel like an athlete, and that kept me going. So did the realization that I was doing better each day. Even when I was sick in bed with a cold or flu and swimming was impossible, I would get up and walk before going back to bed for the day. Exercise was my lifeline, and I could not give that up.

Numinous Experience

One morning while walking and feeling the sweat warm me and seeing the beauty around as the seasons changed, I burst into tears. I was suddenly overcome with the sense of being part of all of the beauty and grandeur—the flowering, the fruiting, even the dying.

It's not so bad to grow old and die, I thought. *I'm part of God's world and God's plan. This is how it works.* That moment of belonging and acceptance was very reassuring to me.

Getting More Involved

The more I walked, the better I got. Even the stiffness in all my joints that had made me feel a hundred years old had gone away. In fact, it felt so good to walk that I decided to enter one of the MS Society walks. It was not a race and most people were ambling along, stopping to view points of interest around the town, or were stopping to eat the food offered at various locations along the way, but just to keep up I found I had to keep moving. The route took me three and a half hours without a stop, but I made it to the end.

Encouraged by my success, I decided to enter a one-mile fun run race two weeks later. Eagerly I started off with the others, but they left me in the dust from the beginning. By the time I reached the first turn, the police officer directing traffic said I would have to walk on the sidewalk because I was so far behind. When I rounded the last turn to the finish line, everyone was gone. Even the time clock had been taken away. I was heart broken. Looking back, I realize how foolish I was to imagine I could keep up and not be part of a group of people like me so we could cheer each other on, but at the time I was still too afraid to talk about having multiple sclerosis to allow myself to get involved with others who had multiple sclerosis, except as a doctor.

At least the next time I entered a fun run race, I made sure that my son was running in the 10K race the same day so I would have a cheering section. This time, pushing myself to the limit, I was not the last one to cross the finish line. The fact that others finishing after me were chatting away and barely strolling along did not matter. My son came in thirty-ninth in a field of hundreds and felt terrible about his poor performance. But for me, coming in so far behind most of the other walkers, the race had been a triumph. How circumstance alters perspective!

Soon after this race, I read a book by one of the famous doctor-runners. He described the joys of running, but he especially stressed winning. I thought, *You don't understand. It's not about winning; it's about running the race!* Several years later, I read an article by the same doctor. He had grown old and had discovered the same thing. He was still running in marathons even though he was no longer among the top runners. He had learned that the joy was simply about being alive and able to complete the goal.

Finding a Mental Image

Near the end of the year of exercise, I went to a Jungian-focused retreat called *Journey in Wholeness.* The participants were asked to think of one word to describe themselves. My first thought was *courageous,* but that made me want to weep. Then I thought of *athlete*! That made me smile and feel strong. Instead of seeing myself as struggling against weakness, I chose to see myself as strong and competent. Mental image is all-important. I could not help but think of my mother and grandmother who were such models of strength while living with pain, and wish I had known then what I know now about the importance of exercise and stretching.

Overdoing It

After a full year of exercise and stretching, I started doing more outdoor activities. On one occasion, birding with friends, I pushed myself too hard. The next day I had so much pain that I could hardly walk. This time, when the pain did not go away, I decided I should see a sports medicine doctor; after all, I was now an athlete.

The doctor took one look at me with my limp and said, "You don't belong here. You need to be at the rehab hospital across the way. For this acute injury, you need to stop exercising for two weeks and just rest."

"No." I said. "I can't stop exercising; I'll get worse. I need your help to keep going."

"Well, you do *sound* like an athlete, anyway," he reluctantly agreed. He shot cortisone into my hip and turned me over to his physical therapist. Fortunately, this PT listened. I told him about all my exercise and stretching routine and explained how important it was for me to keep going, even if I was temporarily injured. "It took me a long time to build up to walking every day for an hour and swimming a mile a day," I told him. "But now, after walking for forty minutes or so, I feel like I could keep going forever. I never felt that good before."

"Sounds like the high runners experience when their endorphins kick in," he said. "I've worked with many people who have multiple sclerosis, but I've never before heard anyone with MS describe that feeling of being able to go on and on."

I laughed and said, "That's probably because people with multiple sclerosis don't exercise enough to get to the point when the endorphins kick in!"

He suggested using ice and shifting the kind of exercise I did until the pain got better, but he did not tell me to stop. That therapist helped a lot. His interest in what I was doing, his guidance about how to get through this acute injury, and his encouragement to trust my judgment was what I really needed. In a matter of weeks, I was better and back to my routine. What a difference it made to get such a positive message.

Still, I had to learn the lesson of not overdoing. Parts of my body are vulnerable because of weakness or past injury. Now, if I overdo—stand too long or walk too far, or spend too long playing the piano or doing glasswork—I set up spasms in my weakened muscles that take time to recover. When I notice the discomfort, I may need to take a break, rest more, do a little stretching, sit for a while, or move around to do everything I want to do. Otherwise, overdoing takes its toll.

Pain Free at Last

In the end, I did swim the fifty miles. It took me seven months, but by the end of that time, I was walking an hour a day and swimming an hour and twelve minutes. It was exhilarating to exercise that long, but the most amazing thing was that I had *no pain.* No pain! No one had told me that if I worked that hard, I could get rid of all the pain! True, if I did not exercise for two or three days, I could tell the old pain was coming back, but as long as I kept going with my program, I had no pain that could not just be walked off or stretched out. With another year of exercising and stretching, the pain no longer came back, even if I did not exercise for days.

No physician or physical therapist had ever told me that if I worked at exercising and stretching that hard, I could *rid myself of the pain altogether* and do away with the depression that had led me to withdraw from my friends and lose interest in doing things. Of course, not all pain can be eliminated through exercise and stretching. Tight muscles and tendons are only one set of factors that cause pain. But they are one source of pain that may be eliminated with persistent exercise and stretching. Even if the major source of pain is something like cancer, addressing the part of the pain made worse by inactivity will improve the situation. And it does not have to take two hours a day. Little bits of exercise and stretching built into one's daily routine can help.

Several doctors had sent me to see physical therapists, but the focus of that therapy had always been on a particular injury or a particular weakness from multiple sclerosis. Even the personal trainers I had hired from time to time to help me expand my program never got beyond a round on the exercise machines. No one saw my need for an overall program or aimed me in that direction, even though athletic training is well understood and is even big business. It seems that once a person is seen as sick, there is very little to get doctors or others to direct them to be physically fit. Many athletes participate in training programs, but until this point I had not realized how important an athletic program is for every person, especially those with physical limitations or depression.

As recently as last year, when Medicare paid for me to spend two weeks in Lakeshore Rehab Hospital following knee replacement surgery because having multiple sclerosis meant I would need more care, the only exercises the physical therapy staff would give me was for the knee itself. It mattered not that I was self-motivated and eager to do more. They had a protocol for each surgery and would do no more than what it called for. Fortunately, the physical therapist I was sent after my return home recognized the importance of all aspects of my attempt to stay fit and responded to all of my questions. She mentioned how much resistance she got most of the time from patients who did not want to move while they hurt. Unless we see fitness as important for all individuals and make movement a part of all medical interventions, we limit our usefulness as physicians facing a challenged population.

Practicing Medicine

My experience with exercise and stretching changed the way I practiced medicine. Never again would I put patients on medication without addressing their lifestyle issues, finding out how they spend their time, and especially how they exercise. And that meant doing more than just saying, "You need to exercise and lose weight." After all, lack of physical activity and changes in weight may be manifestations of a decreased will to live and thus need to be investigated in depth.

I realized that if I, a practicing physician, had been unable to get the help I needed, it would be infinitely more difficult for people to find the way who were not physicians and may not have had the benefits of nurturing care and good role models in youth.

Day-to-Day Activities Are What Count

Statistics show that a certain amount of exercise is needed to decrease the risk of heart disease, cancer, and other debilitating conditions. Hence, everyone needs to exercise a certain amount. But for those with sedentary lifestyles (and that is most Americans today), a daily routine is vital. Certainly, for those with injuries, chronic pain, or a chronic illness that affects function, a systematic program to build strength and endurance—not for a month, not for a year, but for a lifetime of functioning at the maximum—is essential.

Each person living with pain must be his or her own coach; each body is different, and only the one in it can know for sure if rest or stretching or exercise is what is needed at any particular moment. For athlete and couch potato alike, listening to the body is important in deciding what to do next.

When making changes in behavior, like changing exercise or eating habits, it is the small decisions to do a little more (or a little less) over time that matter. It is not the occasional splurge that counts, or the occasional day of rest without exercise; it is *the small decisions, day to day, about food and exercise, creative activity, and being with friends and family that make the difference.* I was fortunate that at this crucial time I was motivated not to gain weight and worked so hard to do better day to day. When motivation is not strong we must find inspiration where we may and keep going. Having a supportive physician or a buddy helps.

The Importance of Listening to the Spirit

While I was fortunate to be motivated to keep going, coming to terms with how I fit into this world made a huge difference to me in the process of my life. It gave me a measure of acceptance that is essential if I am not to get caught up in loss. It also gave me a gift of understanding that I might never have known. And finally, it gave me an element of empathy with others also struggling with what life brought their way. This ultimately led me to seek out opportunities to work with patients with chronic pain who suffered with depression, anxiety, difficulty sleeping, and the loneliness that goes along with all of these. Little did I know what my sojourn as psychiatrist working with medical patients would teach me about spirituality. As we will see, spirituality is more than going to church on Sunday. Spirituality is the essence of the human journey through life.

Hard Times

The connection between emotion and behavior is a complex one. First, on a visit to Montreal to see my boyfriend, he told me, "I don't want to marry someone with an uncertain future." We had walked all over the city earlier that day until I realized I could not keep going. I had been tearful then, but I was dry eyed when he told me. I knew this was the end of our relationship, but instead of dwelling on my loss, I could not help but think about my conversation a few days earlier with a Jewish psychiatrist who had fled Nazi Germany. *How could one man see my soul,* I thought, *while the other, my boyfriend, only see me as a potential burden? Did suffering and loss convey a special ability to see beyond the superficial which a life of success denies?* I wondered.

Within a week, I fell and broke my foot. Was there a connection? Who knows? I had walked for an hour, gone swimming for an hour and twelve minutes, then went to the market and tripped over the sidewalk. Splat! I managed to walk home, but after a nap, I had so much pain and swelling in the foot, I knew I was in trouble. I tried to work the next day, but the pain was too great. I had to wear a cast for six weeks, so I was immobilized.

After six weeks of inactivity, exercise felt like starting at the beginning. *How can they put an athlete in a cast for six weeks and not find a substitute exercise?* I thought after I realized what had happened to me. After that I did exercise almost every day, but I never got back to the level I had achieved during the years before the fall. Still, the lesson I had learned about exercise and stretching has served me well over the years. I know that when I hurt, the first thing is to drink a glass of water and then stretch and exercise the part that hurts. With age or multiple sclerosis, there is arthritis due to wear and tear on the joints, in addition to periodic injuries. Knowing that exercise with stretching is the key to keeping pain at bay keeps me going.

I have also found ways to maintain my fitness level even when I am grounded for one reason or another, as I have been over the years. The answer is doing exercises lying in a bed or sitting in a chair, either with or without machines to make exercising easier. Gradually I have found a routine that accommodates whatever I am able to do at the moment. It is definitely harder if you stop exercising and have to restart from scratch; it is better to keep fit, even while injured.

EMOTION:
THE
KEY
TO
UNDERSTANDING

CHAPTER SIX

EXPANDING MY UNDERSTANDING OF HOW MEDICINE WORKS

Difficult times have helped me to understand better than
before, how infinitely rich and beautiful life is in every
way, and that so many things one goes worrying about
are of no importance whatsoever.
—Isak Dinesen

Although the world is full of suffering, it is full also of
the overcoming of it.
—Helen Keller

At age fifty, I decided to volunteer to work with MS patients. Patients might have had multiple sclerosis for years before a correct diagnosis could be made and often were a mystery for their physicians. This was before MRIs made diagnosing multiple sclerosis far easier. In those days, UAB had an multiple sclerosis clinic to help evaluate patients who came in with a diagnosis of multiple sclerosis, but presented some problem or question for their physicians. In this clinic neurologists from around the state would send questionable cases of multiple sclerosis to the experts at UAB hoping for clarification. They also sent difficult patients with multiple sclerosis who needed special procedures or other help. I thought my expertise with depression and anxiety meant I might have something to offer these patients.

Before my first day in the clinic, I started to worry: *What if seeing what will happen to me in the future is too scary?* As it turned out, seeing patients with severe disease reassured me that even in the most difficult lives, blessings abound. One woman who was unable to move even to feed herself was especially inspiring. She felt blessed to be loved and cared for and was fully engaged with the world around her. I marveled at the resilience of the human spirit.

"I had known my husband for years before I got MS." She told me. "He asked me to marry him when he could see I was getting worse and needed someone to care for me. He has brought a world of friends and good fun to my life. He also built bird feeders for me so that I can watch birds while he's at work. All the birds have such unique personalities." She had come seeking help for her biggest problem—pain from contractures in her legs—but in the midst of such a terrible illness, she had such a positive attitude and was surrounded by love and joy.

Anxiety and Depression: The Pathway to Physical Illness

When I joined the multiple sclerosis clinic staff, I discovered that my approach to patients was strikingly different from that used by the neurologists. The neurologists tended to zero in on physical symptoms, then do an exam to demonstrate what they could find. I, on the other hand would ask what was bothering the patients. That took me in many directions, sometimes finding a physical problem, sometimes uncovering life stresses brought on by the patients' difficulty. Since I accompanied the neurologists during their exams, I noticed that the neurologists tended to see patients as either emotionally upset or physically ill, but not both. I, on the other hand, understood that the most anxious and depressed patients, as well as patients with manifestations of anxiety such as pseudo-symptoms, were *more likely* to have lesions of multiple sclerosis or something else physically wrong. That meant I pushed harder in my search for a physical problem that had yet to be diagnosed if the patient had a manifestations of anxiety or depression.

Time after time, I found evidence of brain involvement from multiple sclerosis in these depressed and anxious patients, often to the amazement of the neurologists who had dismissed the patient as *merely hysterical*. The lesions were not in areas affecting motor function, so they did not show up on the physical exams. Sadly, in multiple sclerosis, patients are *more* likely to have manifestations of anxiety because subcortical areas of the brain may be affected by the multiple sclerosis (resulting in emotional symptoms like anxiety, depression and even mania). In addition patients may be more anxious because they are aware of lesions too small to detect on a physical exam.

Eventually, magnetic resonance imaging (MRI) became routine and did away with a lot of the guesswork in the diagnosis of multiple sclerosis and the resulting physician bias in treating the disease, but findings from MRIs do not address the complex issues involving emotional changes. And emotional complexity is very much an issue today in conditions like chronic pain, which has replaced illnesses like multiple sclerosis for diagnostic confusion and mistrust *because pain still cannot be measured by a test.* Now, as then, physicians tend to compartmentalize the emotional from the physical even though it cannot be done.

As a result of my work in the MS clinic, the head of Neurology came to see me. He had been asked to take over the Department of Psychiatry as well as neurology, but said he would only consider it if I would head up the psychiatry part! Imagine my astonishment. However unfair my earlier firing had been, it was hard not to internalize the feeling of being undesirable. I told him that I would welcome the opportunity to make a difference in the way patients are treated. In the end, the university decided not to combine the departments, but I continued to work with MS patients to help sort out their issues. I felt blessed to be useful and wanted.

Lessons from Afar

After my daughter finished college, I travelled with her to Sao Paulo, Brazil, to visit her violin teacher. Before we left I attended a meeting in Atlanta, wolfing down the available food and peanuts before getting on the plane. By the time I arrived in Sao Paulo seven hours later, I was massively swollen.

Sao Paulo is a beautiful city, but it had so many homeless people, every scrap of land had become occupied. In addition it was no longer safe to go downtown to shop; the symphony had closed the year before because of patrons being assaulted; and women did not go outside without a group or a man. Everyone lived behind walls or fences. Cars were never left on the streets for fear of looting. I could not help but wonder if this was the future for us in America as well if we did not do a better job fighting poverty.

The violin teacher gave lessons every day, so while she taught, I stayed in the bedroom, my legs against the wall reading books. To my delight I found Jean Carper's book, *Food–Your Miracle Medicine* which opened my eyes to the role of nutrition in health and disease. Carper talked about the horrors of the American diet and the diseases it caused. She also explored the healing properties of vegetables and fruits along with omega-3-oils from fatty fishes. There were several chapters that dealt with medical conditions whose inflammation and resulting pain were directly related to diet. I was horrified. I had been a doctor for more years than I wanted to admit, and this was new thinking for me. I had been struggling with weight off and on, going on one diet program after another, but no one had mentioned the whole concept of specifically what we eat and what it does to us. Diets had been about reducing calories, substituting lower calorie foods, not about healthy eating.

Brazil had wonderful fruits and we had a wide selection for breakfast every morning, some I had not even heard of before. I dreaded the trip home because I had such trouble with swelling on the trip down. But this time I had no problem I assumed because of what I had been eating. I resolved to eat nine fruits and vegetables a day, and fish three times a week to get omega 3 oils. At least that way I would not eat as much of the unhealthy foods.

Finding New Teaching Strategies

On the trip home my daughter suggested I join her at the International Simulation and Gaming Association (ISAGA) meeting at the University of Michigan in the fall. I was delighted to attend to learn how to use educational simulations in my teaching with medical students and patients. The first educational game I developed I called, *The Pain Game.* It gave participants an opportunity to make various decisions about their care so they could experience the outcome of making those particular choices. For example, patients with back pain could choose physical therapy, bed rest or their usual activities. Those with activity, whether physical therapy or the usual ones, did well. Only the person who took to bed without any exercise did poorly. A patient with rheumatoid arthritis could choose to avoid nightshade vegetables (tomatoes, potatoes, peppers, or eggplant) or suffer the consequences. I used this educational game with medical students and nurses as well as with patients who had various causes of chronic pain.

Another educational program I developed for patients was called *Binge Buster.* After investigating processed foods in the market I realized they were all aimed at making money, not enhancing nutrition. The educational game was to reinforce choices at the market based on reading food labels, and choosing items closest to nature without additives like sugars and preservatives like nitrites that prolong shelf life, but not human life.

CHAPTER SEVEN

THE STORY OF INBORN
ANXIOUSNESS AND PAIN

The greatest mistake in the treatment of diseases is that
there are physicians for the body and physicians for the
soul, although the two cannot be separated.
—Plato

Even as a youngster, I knew I was an anxious person. Always a good student and good at sports and piano, I still was fearful of failure and made bargains with God to protect me. During my twenties, I started having migraine headaches. In my thirties, I began having episodes of extreme fatigue that came on suddenly in the middle of the afternoon, when I just had to lie down no matter what I was doing. When the fatigue did not immediately go away, I went to see an internist, who ran numerous tests. All the results came back normal, except for one thing: I had mitral valve prolapse (MVP), a floppy heart valve. The doctor did not know if it had anything to do with my fatigue symptoms, but mitral valve prolapse had only recently been described, and many doctors still did not believe the syndrome of mitral valve prolapse really existed.

Mitral valve prolapse was first described by Dr. Cecil Coghlan at a clinic in the University of Alabama School of Medicine (UASOM). The connection between MVP and other conditions was first discovered in the 1970s in patients with hypoglycemia (low blood sugar). In the process of obtaining a routine history and performing some tests on a group of patients with low blood sugar, doctors at UASOM found that the patients tended to have a number of other conditions in common. They had migraine headaches, MVP, irritable bowel syndrome (IBS), temporomandibular joint problems (TMJ), postural hypotension (drop in blood pressure upon standing up) leading to dizzy spells, and fainting spells. The doctors also realized that after ingesting a sugar load, these patients' blood sugar levels were no lower than those of other patients after a sugar load. The difference was that *these patients could feel when their blood sugar started to drop.* As their blood sugar dropped below a certain level, their heart rates increased and they began to sweat and feel faint. The symptoms and treatments for mitral valve prolapse were worked out and written up by Dr. Coghlan and his nurse, Lynn Fredricks.[14]

In the early 1980s, I attended a meeting to discuss this syndrome. The speakers revealed more conditions associated with mitral valve prolapse in this same group of patients: sleep disorders, attention deficit disorders, and even some fertility problems.

After that I began seeing a number of patients with mitral valve prolapse syndrome because they tended to develop symptoms of depression and panic attacks under stress; they also tended to be sensitive to the side effects of medicines and therefore failed to take medications as prescribed. These people have what might be described as a sensitive nervous system.

Many of these individuals had been ridiculed by their physicians and others who saw them as *neurotic,* a word used to describe silly women without any real complaints and now used pejoratively to dismiss patients' symptoms. However, I found that many of my patients were men, who were equally mystified by their various symptoms. These patients are anxious by nature and can feel the changes in their bodies when something is not right.

Many had been to several doctors and even different specialists, looking for answers. Young persons who have chest pain from a panic attack often go to the emergency room, because they are afraid they

---

[14] Lynn Fredericks, "When Panic Attacks," *MVP Update: The Mitral Valve Prolapse Center of Alabama Newsletter* (Birmingham, AL: Montclair Medical Center, 1993), 5.

are having a heart attack. Those who are depressed might seek medical attention and complain of nerves or fatigue or multiple pains, and although medical doctors may run a few tests to rule out something they consider medically serious, they often think the tests are a waste of time. It is only since depression has been recognized as a serious contributor to increased mortality from heart attacks that physicians in general have become more respectful (and, to be fair, more knowledgeable) about depression and anxiety and of the importance of identifying a sensitive nervous system with the patient so he or she can be guided in the right direction. Patients with sensitive nervous systems may have a number of symptoms under stress that may otherwise be difficult for a physician to identify.

Patients with Mitral Valve Prolapse Seek Help for Depression

Mary Tate was a woman in her late thirties who had four children. "I'm a very sick person," she told me as she sat down the first day in my office. She rattled off the terms she had heard from her physicians: "I have migraine headaches, temporomandibular joint pain, mitral valve prolapse, irritable bowel syndrome, chronic anxiety with panic disorder, dysthymic disorder, that's depression, sleep apnea, attention deficit disorder, and dysautonomia."

"What have your doctors told you about how these relate to one another?" I asked. I wanted to see how much Mary knew about her condition and whether doctors were making the connection for her.

"They haven't," Mary said. She had seen a number of doctors and had been run through multiple tests, all with negative results. Different doctors had prescribed the many pills she was taking: a neurologist for her migraine headaches, a dentist for her jaw pain from TMJ, a cardiologist for her chest pain from mitral valve prolapse, a gastroenterologist for her stomach pain from irritable bowel syndrome, doctors at a sleep center for her sleep apnea, and a psychiatrist for her anxiety, panic attacks, and depression.

"The doctors say they can't cure me," she lamented. She was a young woman, and she was applying for disability benefits because she was sick all the time and, with all the medicine, often too sleepy to function. When I asked her what stress she was under, she burst into tears and poured out her story. Once she finished talking, she felt better.

One of the ways I found to help people who have symptoms of a sensitive nervous system is to demystify what is happening to them. So I told this story: "If a tiger were to come through that door, even if you have a sensitive nervous system and I do not, we would both react. Our blood pressure and pulse would go up, and we would both break out into a sweat. But your system would go bonkers." At this point Mary nodded, because she knew well her typical response to stress. "The problem is," I told her, "life is filled with lots of little—and some not-so-little—tigers. Some tigers come from the outside; they might be family problems or financial problems. Others come from inside, like anger or fear. Also, some foods such as sugar and white flour, caffeine, and alcohol will trigger a sensitive nervous system. But there are activities that can counteract these tigers, such as regular daily exercise, daily meditation or stress management exercises, problem solving, and talking out difficulties. A sensitive nervous system is not a disease, but it sure can make you feel sick if it is not managed well."

From there, we talked about sensitivity to the side effects of medicines and determined that she should probably take less than the regular amount—or even stop medicines altogether when they made her feel worse (unless she was taking antibiotics or steroids that had to be full dose). Her doctor had given her medication but had not mentioned any of the activities she could do to help herself.

Sensitive Nervous Systems Run in Families

"What about your relatives?" I asked her. "Do any of them have these kinds of symptoms?"

She nodded her head. "My mother and two of my sisters do. I don't know about the rest, because we don't tend to talk about such things."

"So, as you can see, these kinds of problems run in families," I underscored for her. After that, I inquired about symptoms of depression, anxiety, and panic attacks (I already had details about symptoms from her intake questionnaire) and then described how these relate to sensitive nervous systems. When I explained to her how all her symptoms fit together and what she could do about them, she looked vastly relieved.

"Why hasn't anyone told me this before?" she asked. Instead of feeling helpless and out of control, she now had a direction. It would not make her symptom free, but it would at least help her manage her symptoms and her life.

Because I have seen medical patients for depression for most of my professional life, I have seen this scenario played out over and over, but not all with such favorable results. Some patients, once on a disability track, do not want to hear anything else until they get their check. Others feel so overwhelmed that they cannot give up the sick-role niche they have adopted.

This is one place where physicians play a crucial role: they can either promote disability and the sense of being really sick, or they can help people manage their lives well. This is an example of how the medical model and the story it conveys about a patient's condition make all the difference, both in how the patient is treated by the medical profession and in how he or she manages the condition in day-to-day living.

The sensitive nervous system condition, now called neuroendocrine-dysautonomia (NED), is a fairly recently understood phenomenon. Although physicians have known about some aspects of the problem for years, they have mistrusted other parts of the syndrome because they could not demonstrate a cause on any medical tests. The symptoms were considered functional rather than an illness. One of my medical colleagues was among the greatest skeptics. "I don't believe mitral valve prolapse really exists," he said. "That woman is just neurotic!" Since being anxious can cause physical symptoms, this might have been an attempt at defining the source of this patient's problem, but generally when physicians and others use "neurotic" in this way, it constitutes a put-down. And while put-downs may disguise uncertainty or ignorance on the part of the doctor, when the *neurotic* is a patient, the lack of understanding comes too often at the patient's expense. Later, this same doctor found that he and members of his family had neuroendocrine dysautonomia!

How Does This All Fit Together?

I first began to see how a sensitive nervous system works when I heard an address about inborn personality characteristics at a psychiatric meeting. Anxiousness it turns out is an inborn characteristic. The other inborn characteristics, by the way, are introversion/extroversion, agree-ableness, openness, and conscientiousness.[15] Each of these personality characteristics can be measured on a continuum from a little to a lot and varies from person to person, and while these characteristics can be modified through influences in the environment such as training, educa-tion and life experience they represent fundamental characteristics im-mutable over time.

Inborn, of course, means one is born that way. It is part of our make-up like having red hair or a turned up nose. It can be altered to some extent through influences in the environment. For anxiousness that means planning ahead or daily exercise and meditation to promote the calming effect of the parasympathetic nervous system, but anxiousness is always a factor that has to be dealt with. Inborn also implies that the condition runs in families. Looking back, I saw that anxiousness had run in my own family for generations. Early in my medical career I learned that some people are so anxious by nature that they might need to be on lifelong medication, but here was one specific reason: they are born with a sensitive nervous system.

Interestingly, the susceptibility to addiction or alcoholism that also runs in families is probably at the opposite end of the spectrum of in-born-anxiousness. Addicts tend to have under rather than overstimulated nervous systems. Addicts look for ways to get revved up, while people

---

[15] Inborn means we are prone to certain characteristic by nature. With education and effort we may mitigate the effect these in-born characteristics have on our lives, but these factors are part of our make-up.

with sensitive nervous systems want to keep things under control. They are less likely to experiment with drugs or do risky things. They may drink or overuse tranquilizers to calm their nerves, but they do not like to feel out of control themselves.

The concept of a sensitive nervous system is still under appreciated, however, leaving patients with neuroendocrine dysautonomia misunderstood and mistreated. Medical residents rotating through my service in the past few years have told me over and over that they have never been exposed to the concept. Why not? Currently in medicine, and even more commonly in psychiatry, each cluster of symptoms is defined as a disease or illness; whereas other diseases or illnesses that occur along with it are described as *comorbid* conditions. This clustering began as an attempt to pigeon-hole similar conditions for the purpose of research. But rapidly took on a legitimacy of its own, which often fails to be useful to patients who tend to resist pigeonholing.

In the case of neuroendocrine dysautonomia, a rheumatologist treats fibromyalgia, a painful condition involving the muscles. A cardiologist treats mitral valve prolapse, which often presents as chest pain. A neurologist treats migraine headaches. A gastroenterologist treats irritable bowel syndrome (spastic colon). A sleep center treats the sleep disorders. A psychiatrist treats the depression, anxiety, ADD, and panic attacks, and the gynecologist and chiropractor treat the infertility. Each diagnosis labels the others' symptoms as co-morbid or co-occurring conditions. It is a true case of the blind men describing the elephant. But here, the more reasonable diagnosis, because it identifies the cause, is neuroendocrine dysautonomia (NED) or sensitive nervous system, just as the diagnosis of reason in a drinker with pancreatitis, cirrhosis of the liver, broken bones, and dementia is alcoholism.

Failure to recognize neuroendocrine dysautonomia as an affirmative diagnosis, not the one left over when everything else has been eliminated, is part of the problem. Identifying neuroendocrine dysautonomia is easy and cost-effective (there are no fancy tests needed), and it makes all the difference to the patient. Patients may have many of the conditions associated with it, or only one. Although the treatment for individual disorders may be different, the management is the same for all. The next example demonstrates part of the problem.

Susan Johnson was referred to me for depression and panic attacks. She had all the diagnoses that represent neuroendocrine dysautonomia: severe headaches several times a week, stomach pain and diarrhea, and chest pains that made her feel as though she were going to die (panic attacks). She was pessimistic about ever being able to have a reasonable life, because her life was already highly stressful. I told her how all her symptoms fit together and started her on an antidepressant, daily exercise (walking), and breathing exercises for stress management. I made her an appointment to come back to talk some more.

When she did return, she told this story: She had gone to the emergency room of another hospital with a panic attack and was admitted for some tests. First, she was seen by a neurologist for her headaches; he did an MRI of her head. The gastroenterologist performed a colonoscopy to try to determine the reason for her abdominal pain and diarrhea, and the cardiologist used cardiac catheterization to determine the cause of her chest pains. All the test results were normal. The ER doctors told her she had irritable bowel syndrome, mitral valve prolapse, and migraine headaches, with depression and panic attacks—all of which she had known before she went!

Aside from the costs and risks associated with unnecessary tests, the biggest problem for patients like Mrs. Johnson is that they are naturally anxious—and being treated in this way tends to make them more anxious. As one patient said to me, "If the doctor didn't think there was something bad wrong, he wouldn't have done the test!"

Doctors tend to feel they have to rule out other diagnoses, particularly life-threatening ones. This is part of doctor training. Doctors may even give the patient several medications to control specific symptoms, yet fail to educate him or her about the overall problem and how it can be managed. Because people with a sensitive nervous system may constitute as many as 20 to 25 percent of the population, this means a lot of unnecessary tests and over treatment if neuroendocrine dysautonomia is not identified.

People with neuroendocrine dysautonomia are sensitive to the side effects of many medications. Most of the time, patients get used to or develop tolerance to the side effects; that is, the side effects go away. But for patients with a sensitive nervous system, physicians need to start medicines out at a much lower dose and build up gradually, so the side effects can wear off by increments.

Once individuals realize they have this condition, they can do a number of things to help themselves not to feel sick and out of control all the time. Patients are more in control of doing what they need to do to live well.

Patients with Neuroendocrine Dysautonomia: Getting the Story Right

The Reverend Mr. Scott Cole was referred to me for treatment of depression; he had full-blown neuroendocrine dysautonomia syndrome. He had been given multiple diagnoses and believed that he was a very sick man. Formerly a missionary for his church, he had had to return home because he was sick all the time. He felt abandoned by God and looked down on by his fellow priests. He had a sack full of medicines from different doctors, had tried every antidepressant, and was feeling worse and worse.

As I learned more about his particular symptoms, I told him the story of Mrs. Johnson. As he listened and answered my questions, he felt reassured that he understood what was wrong and that he could do something about his problem. Human beings have tremendous resilience and resolve once they know what to do. "So what can I do to manage my sensitive nervous system?" he asked.

My advice to him ran something like this: "First, and perhaps most important, is to do things that give you some control over your nervous system so it does not have control over you. *Regular daily exercise switches off an overactive sympathetic nervous system.* This exercise can be slow, but it needs to be consistent, and ideally it should last forty to sixty minutes per day.

"Using *breathing exercises* to disengage an overactive sympathetic nervous system is another way to regain some control. You can do relaxation exercises like focused breathing, mindfulness meditation, or guided imagery. These disciplines help you train your mind to let go of stress and to dissociate from things you can't handle. Prayer can help as well."

"You should avoid sweets, caffeine, alcohol, and other substances that upset your system. Sugar, white flour, and highly processed foods are more likely to stimulate a drop in blood sugar that you can feel." Even though I had a handout for him that summarized the points, I noticed that he took out a pad and paper to make notes.

I continued, "Learning to deal with your emotions in general is important, as well as working out specific problems so they don't turn your stress into physical symptoms. We all get angry, but how we deal with anger can make the difference between becoming anxious and depressed or putting ourselves in a better position. Some people blame themselves when they get angry, while some blame others when there is a problem. Getting enough information about what is really happening and bouncing it off someone else is an important way to sort out events. Avoid making assumptions or guesses about another's behavior without enough particulars. Ruminating or imagining a dialogue is a sure way to stay ignorant about what is going on. Involve the other person. If you understand that person better as a result, you may have a better friend. Or you may learn enough to run far away from him or her."

"You know the old saying: If you meet a man who knows and knows he knows, learn from him. If you meet a man who knows but doesn't know he knows, wake him up. If you meet a man who doesn't know and knows he doesn't know, teach him, but if you meet a man who doesn't know and doesn't know he doesn't know, get as far away from him as you can. To know which is which, *you have to get enough information.*

"Finally, it is important for you to know that just because you have a sensitive nervous system does not mean you are sick or mentally ill; neither does it mean you have an unstable personality. Be aware that the medication can make you worse if you don't watch out. So find a professional who understands your system to help you work out symptoms and problems as they come along. That is part of taking care of yourself.

Finally, be aware that a sensitive nervous system can put you in touch with the pathos of life, which can lead you to become a wiser person."

Autoimmune Disease:
Its Connection with a Sensitive Nervous System

For years I had known that autoimmune diseases ran in my family. Rheumatoid arthritis, multiple sclerosis, even Hashimoto's thyroiditis had appeared in different family members, but I had never made the connection between these conditions and neuroendocrine dysautonomia until I began seeing it in my patients.

One day in the mid-nineties, after interviewing several patients with neuroendocrine dysautonomia who had autoimmune diseases, I called a colleague at the Mitral Valve Prolapse Center at the Baptist Medical Center in Birmingham to see if he knew what this connection was all about. He explained that patients with neuroendocrine dysautonomia are more apt to suppress their immune systems under stress, which sets them up to develop autoimmune diseases. Are they the only ones who get autoimmune diseases? No, of course not; people who do not have neuroendocrine dysautonomia can get them. But, once more, if the connection between neuroendocrine dysautonomia and autoimmune diseases is not recognized, treating stress in the sensitive individual does not receive the priority it deserves to prevent the development or worsening of autoimmune disease. While I cannot say that my discovery of exercise to recover from pain stopped my multiple sclerosis from progressing, exercise contributed immeasurably to my ability to remain functional and to live a full life.

Medical Stories Are Important to the Patient

This is why finding the right story for patients is crucial to their survival so they know how best to manage their lives. Just giving a diagnosis, which may be devastating in itself, without showing the patient how best to manage the illness within the context of their life, may not equip him or her to do what is necessary to survive. Medical stories play an important role in how physicians approach patients and whether they give patients something to act on or not. In the area of pain management, surgical and medical interventions are an important part of the story, but not the whole tale. Unless the message involves the behavioral and emotional aspects of the pain problem, the patient may get worse rather than better. These aspects of modern treatment are often addressed by approaches best defined as prevention, complementary and alternative medicine, or even psychotherapy.

CHAPTER EIGHT

PHYSICAL PROBLEMS GET CONFUSED WITH UNCONSCIOUS RESPONSES TO ANXIETY

*It is more important to know what sort of person has a
disease than to know what sort of disease a person has.*
—William Osler, MD

Nowhere does finding the right story—that is, understanding the connection between physical symptoms and responses to stress and anxiety—become more important than when neuroendocrine dysautonomia (NED), mitral valve prolapse (MVP), and other physical problems get confused with unconscious responses to anxiety. I used to say that my favorite patients were those who had already been to a number of other physicians without success, because *I always knew what was wrong with them before I saw them*! I knew they all had something physically wrong, perhaps already known, perhaps not, and that they all had some depression and/or some manifestation of anxiety, or an unconscious defense against anxiety. Sometimes my role was to look beyond the symptom to find the underlying physical problem, but sometimes that was already known and the problem lay in responses of anxiety, depression, or substance abuse.

Mrs. Jackie Ray was a young woman referred to me by a neurologist in the emergency room. The neurologist said the patient was paralyzed, but not from a physical cause: it was a pseudo-paralysis, meaning that there was no muscle weakness; the inability to move was caused by extensor and flexor muscles contracting at the same time. This kind of paralysis is an unconscious defense against anxiety, but the neurologist did not know what the patient was anxious about.

The story was this: Jackie Ray had been having spells of paralysis off and on for over nine months and had been unable to work because of them. She had already been to an internist, two neurologists, a psychiatrist, and a sleep center without finding the answer. Each had seen something not covered by their specialty and had referred the patient to someone else. She had a history of severe headaches, usually on the third day of her period, which had been diagnosed by the neurologist as migraines. She suffered from depression and from episodes of pseudo-paralysis that represented anxiety, but she had no apparent stress in her life to account for this. The only negative thing in her life was that she had been unable to get pregnant, but she and her husband had a good marriage and had come to terms with this. The anxiety symptoms provided no apparent benefit to her. She worked because she liked to, not because she had to, and she was not applying for disability, even though she had been unable to work for nine months.

While doing her physical exam, I noticed that she had some drop in blood pressure when she stood up, and although I did not hear a murmur or a click in her heart, I thought she might have mitral valve prolapse and sent her for an evaluation with a cardiologist. She did indeed have mitral valve prolapse, but the cardiologist sent back a note saying, "The mitral valve prolapse is not the cause of her symptoms."

At this point, I went back and reviewed with Jackie when her episodes of paralysis had begun. It turned out that she had been working in a warehouse in the middle of the summer, running up and down the stairs, when she began to have the spells. I could imagine that in the middle of the hot summer, without air conditioning, she was sweating and making her blood pressure drop even more. The attacks of pseudo-paralysis were actually protecting her from blacking out.

Once Jackie realized what the problem was, the pseudo-paralytic episodes stopped. We treated her low blood pressure with support stockings and medicines, and she was encouraged to exercise regularly and keep her salt and water intake up by replacing the salt she lost sweating with a beverage containing salt.

On her own, she found another job that allowed her to manage her condition better; she was able to take a few days off if she went through a bad period and needed more rest. There were no compensation issues related to her previous job (that is, she was not trying to get disability benefits), and when she returned to me over the next several years, I understood more about issues related to and how such symptoms affected this patient and many others.

Jackie had virtually all the symptoms related to neuroendocrine dysautonomia. This patient's highly creative ways to cope with her personal and work lives, once she understood the relationship between her neuroendocrine dysautonomia and the attacks of paralysis underscore the importance of giving patients a story they can use to make sense of their lives, not just a diagnosis and medications. *Diagnoses help doctors organize their thinking, but they are merely constructs that may not enable the patient to make the changes that will help them do better.* Diagnostic labels are sometimes helpful, but sometimes they miss the big picture. The doctor who ran the mitral valve prolapse test said that mitral valve prolapse was not the cause of Jackie's symptoms, but what he failed to recognize was the connection between symptoms of anxiety (pseudo-symptoms) and the physical disorder giving rise to the anxiety.

Over and over, patients were sent to me by their primary care physicians with a diagnosis of hysteria, neurosis, or nerves, only to have me find that they had as-yet unidentified physical problems. My introduction to this state of affairs started when I was in training.

Joe Brown, a workman, was sent to psychiatry because of hysterical spells. He had come to the emergency room saying he had tetanus, but his spells did not appear consistent with that diagnosis. When I first saw him, he was sitting with difficulty, and as I watched, his body became rigid as a board with one spasm after another. Each time his body stiffened, he would throw his arms over his head. He should have been in tremendous pain, but he seemed unconcerned.

The psychiatry professor showing us the patient pointed to the posturing and announced, "This is a case of grand hysteria." I watched with amazement the strange movements and marveled at the seeming disconnect between this man's writhing and his emotional reaction to it–a characteristic of hysteria, but not tetanus. After seeing us, he was observed for a while, given a tranquilizer, and sent home. Three days later, I learned he had reappeared in the emergency room. By then, even the first-year students could see he had tetanus! I never found out what happened to Joe Brown after that, but delay in identifying the medical problem surely was not to his benefit.

Hysteria, now called *conversion disorder*, is characterized by the presence of bogus symptoms—or pseudo-symptoms, as they are called—symptoms that cannot be caused by damaged nerves.[16] Because the symptoms are not caused by damage to the brain or nervous system, hysteria had a bad name. It was thought by many to represent fakery and malingering and to be a sign of weakness. In the early days of my training, it was thought to affect the feebleminded and women disproportionately.

Freud and others recognized that the primary benefit of the hysterical symptom to the patient was to shift the focus away from the source of the anxiety. He also recognized that a secondary benefit to the sufferer was the receipt of care from family, doctors, and others. This *secondary gain,* as it was called, led physicians to see the behavior as manipulative and added to the physician's suspicions of the patient.

We now know that hysteria or conversion symptoms are a response to anxiety that works by removing the subject from awareness of the danger and creating symptoms that need medical care and support. It occurs more often in those with brain damage or illnesses that affect the nervous system and those with severe medical issues and should never be dismissed as malingering. Although insight into the meaning of hysteria has grown over the years, many prejudices against it remain and continue to make evaluation and treatment difficult. Joe Brown had

---

[16] Other examples of hysterical, conversion, or pseudo-symptoms: A patient may be unable to see, though the optic nervous system is intact, or be unable to move, not from muscular weakness, but because the muscles that extend the limb and those that bend it are both contracting at once. Seizures or spasms can occur that look different from those caused by damage to the nervous system.

shown me that hysterical symptoms are not simple and that they *demand further investigation of what is threatening* the patient.

The next patient I saw with the diagnosis of hysteria, Mrs. Mary Thomas, was admitted to me on the psychiatric ward. Mary had been bedridden, unable to walk for so long that she had permanent contractures in her legs. Her physical deformity was severe. This should have been very painful, but she appeared unconcerned. Hysteria was the assumed cause of her inability to walk, because her first symptom appeared about the time she and her husband were having problems and had talked of divorce.

This secondary gain, using physical problems to exact an advantage, was considered the hallmark of the diagnosis of hysteria, and Mary's dependence on her husband was supposed to be a clear indication of that secondary gain. Even Mary herself stated confidently that if it had not been for her hysteria, her husband would have left her years before.

Fresh from my experience with Joe's tetanus, I was prepared to find more than hysteria as the cause of Mary's symptoms. As it turned out, her spinal fluid showed an elevation of IgG protein. Mary had an undiagnosed case of multiple sclerosis. For years physicians had called her problem hysteria because they *could not find anything on a test.* This often happens to patients in pain when the pain is greater than the doctor expects, but that is just the doctor's guess, often wrong.

On the other hand, this patient might have had symptoms of hysteria *in addition* to the multiple sclerosis. Perhaps this is because *hysteria is seen in the presence of a physical problem,* which may or may not have been recognized by the patient or the treating physician. Mrs. Thomas also had symptoms of depression, which she tried very hard to hide, since depression was considered a shameful condition in those days. Treating her depression with medication and helping her see that the source of her difficulty was multiple sclerosis—not that she was a weak person—gave her some relief.

Not long after that, Mrs. Lois Cook came to see me in the clinic. Years before, I had treated Lois for depression and alcoholism. Lois also had multiple sclerosis and had just spent six weeks in the hospital because of pain and paralysis. Her doctors had told her they did not know how long it would be before she would have this problem again. She was terrified that her multiple sclerosis was getting worse. She hurt all the time and had more difficulty getting around. According to her chart, she had had a hysterical paralysis, or pseudo-paralysis, so her doctors did not think the paralysis was due to MS. That prompted me to ask her how long it had been since she had had a new symptom from MS. It had been more than fifteen years.

"Good," I said. "That means your disease has not progressed in fifteen years." Then I asked her how often she had symptoms like the ones that sent her to the hospital and what brought them on. She said that those particular symptoms were brought on by a relapse in her drinking, fights with her husband, and a feeling of not getting enough support at home. She also had symptoms of depression. "Wonderful," I said. "Now you know what you can do to address these particular spells."

I restarted her on medicine for depression, sent her back to Alcoholics Anonymous, and encouraged her to seek marital therapy with her husband. Most of all, I urged her to plan her life so that she had more support: to take regular rests, exercise and stretch every day, plan time for fun, get help around the house, and plan a backup system for when she felt overwhelmed or when she needed more support. She went away delighted, because she no longer felt so helpless and could do something to cut down on the spells of paralysis. Hysterical symptoms blind the patient to what is going on, but once patients identify the source of the anxiety, they can usually find ways to cope with their situations.

This experience taught me that *doctors do not always investigate emotional symptoms in the same way they do physical symptoms*; that is, they do not ask the questions as I had done with this patient that would allow them to sort out the cause of the anxious symptom as they would have done with any physical symptom.

In addition, I recognized that pseudo-neurological, or hysterical, symptoms are a manifestation of anxiety seen most commonly in patients with organic disease. In truth, *I have never seen a patient with pseudo-symptoms who did not also have something physically wrong*. The physical symptom might be relatively minor, like a limp from an old leg injury. Sometimes the physical symptom is known to the patient and the doctor, and sometimes it needs to be found. The failure of doctors to understand that pseudo-symptoms are a manifestation of anxiety often interferes with their ability to offer helpful treatment and leads to patients' increased disability and fear. *Furthermore, a physician's tendency to misunderstand the symptom, call the psychiatrist, and look with suspicion on patients' motives interferes with the doctor-patient relationship and prevents the doctor from becoming an ally.*

The patient's apparent lack of concern about what is happening is one of the cardinal signs of a pseudo-symptom. The person is not concerned because there is a disconnect between conscious awareness and the body. This is akin to the emotional numbing or failure to experience intense emotion associated with a traumatic event. This is just one of the creative brain's tools to protect us from getting overwhelmed by circumstances. Most of the time, these dissociative phenomena help bridge the events of day to day life seamlessly. That is, neither the individual nor those around them are aware that something is wrong. Dissociative events only become a problem when they take over the functioning of the whole individual, as in global amnesia, which is rare.

However, my experience with conversion disorders, and even my residency in psychiatry, did not prepare me to understand the essence of anxiety and its role in our lives or how our belief systems can support us or get us into trouble.

CHAPTER NINE

UNRAVELING THE MYSTERY OF ANXIETY

It is a man's own mind, not his enemy or foe, that lures
him to evil ways.
—Buddha

My first exposure to psychiatry was during my sophomore rotation in medical school. Here, neuroses and personality disorders were presented to us as mental illnesses or disorders of the mind. Imagine my horror when I found I could identify with something in every single category. What could this mean?

My residency training in psychiatry was not much more illuminating when it came to the neuroses or anxiety disorders. I learned that *hysteria*, a clearly pejorative term, was more common in women and the feebleminded, but the primary emphasis was not on what it meant to the patient, but on *secondary gain*, the hall mark of hysteria, as the patient's way to manipulate the doctor and the system. Since secondary gain was hard to distinguish from malingering, physicians were very suspicious of anyone exhibiting hysterical symptoms. I had no idea at the time that the so-called *neuroses* were just manifestations of anxiety that *took the patient to the doctor* and that the word neurotic, so often applied to women in a disparaging way, merely means, *anxious*. It was not until the 1980s that I found a comprehensive explanation that made sense.

At that time, I was taking part in Physicians for Social Responsibility (PSR), a group committed to recognizing the mistake of waging nuclear war. Physicians for Social Responsibility came together initially to address the unworkable civil defense plans the government had developed in response to the threat of nuclear war. Physicians for Social Responsibility took the position that, instead, we needed to take steps to prevent the use of nuclear weapons completely. In 1985 PSR received a Nobel Peace Prize for these efforts.

As a psychiatrist in this organization, my job was to talk about the psychology of the nuclear age, how fear affects decision making and rational planning, and what the threat of nuclear annihilation was doing to us individually and as a society. I wanted to answer the questions, "How do policy makers come up with a survival plan that represents pure fantasy?" What I learned changed forever how I looked at patients and how I understood their strengths and weaknesses. It also changed how I looked at myself.

Finding the Answers

I knew that each personality type evaluates the world from a different perspective, but two factors that affect everyone's thinking about the world involves, first, the unconscious defense mechanisms we all use to ward off that anxiety and second, the layers of beliefs that we absorb from the culture.

Unconscious Defenses against Anxiety

The most helpful discussion of the defense mechanisms I found was Dr. George Vaillant's book, *Adaptation to Life*. This book discusses the Grant Study at Harvard which examined the healthiest people they could find.[17] One parameter researchers thought might reflect psychological health was how an individual used unconscious defenses to manage anxiety. These defenses were first described by Sigmund Freud in the nineteenth century and then expanded upon by his daughter, Anna Freud, and others. While there is not complete agreement about what

---

[17] George E. Vaillant, *Adaptation to Life* (USA: Atheneum Publishing, Inc., 1977).

the defenses are, many defense mechanisms do not overlap and have been confirmed by numerous researchers.

For purposes of this project, the Grant Study divided the defense mechanisms into four categories: mature defenses, neurotic or anxious defenses, immature defenses, and psychotic defenses. Mature defenses are what we call coping mechanisms like humor, helping others, artistic expression, planning ahead and getting on with the business of the day. These defenses bind us to others, which helps in difficult times. Neurotic or anxious defenses include rationalization, intellectualization, obsessions, phobias, reaction formation (doing the opposite as the value is reversed) and the pseudo-neurologic symptoms we have already discussed. These symptoms tend to be benign or may *take us to the doctor for support.* Immature defenses are those we associate with youth or personality disorders because they tend to get the user into trouble. They include things like passive aggressive behavior, acting without thinking through the consequences, blaming others, hypochondriasis and fantasy. Depressed individuals using self defeating behavior may use these defenses as well. (See Appendix *A*). Psychotic defenses like delusions and hallucinations are only present if someone becomes physically or mentally ill, but *even the healthiest people have some mature defenses, some immature defenses, and many anxious defenses.*

The important feature of the defense mechanisms is that they are all *unconscious or semi-conscious*; that is, no one chooses when to use which defense. They are automatic reactions that affect *everyone.* You cannot distinguish between black and white, rich and poor, males and females. Everyone has them. And *they all distort reality to some extent, even the mature defenses.* Everyone uses more immature defenses under stress. As we grow older, we shift away from immature defenses toward more mature defenses, unless there is brain damage or the brain is affected by illness or drugs. But even young people use some mature defenses, and older people some immature ones. Which defense we use at any one time is determined in part by heredity, in part by the seriousness of the threat, and in part by our stage of maturation in life.

As for psychotic defenses, we tend to think of psychosis as being part of severe mental illness like schizophrenia, but it behooves us to remember that anyone may be affected by psychotic defenses in a medical setting where everyone is anxious and as many as 40 percent may be disoriented by infections, chemical imbalances, medication, and a host of other factors related to medical illness, or medical treatment. In this situation any change in behavior or psychiatric symptom must be considered to be part of a medical illness and evaluated as such. Failure to do so may be fatal to the patient.

Lessons from the Defense Mechanisms

When I learned about defense mechanisms, I thought, *What a laugh! All those years I worried that there was something wrong with me when I could identify with symptoms of the neuroses, and it turns out that I'm just a human being!* I also realized that my patients, like me, were just struggling with life, doing the best they could in a world that does not always operate according to our plan.

Life seems to bring about a maturation of defenses for many, which is perhaps related to the increased number of obligations and relationships we cannot get out of. In fact, obligation seems to be the *single most important factor* in maturation. (Is that why we grow up with our children and mature with aging parents?) Psychotherapy which involves a committed relationship, is another powerful tool for encouraging the maturation of defenses.

Defense Mechanisms Give Rise to Cultural Illusions

Defense mechanisms can give rise to illusions that can manifest on a local or even a national level when groups of people embrace the same defensive shifts. The fantasy that we could survive all-out nuclear war was one of these. Cultural illusions can also become institutionalized in the language, or passed on to others in the culture through education (including professional education), religion, the media, or the internet.

Exposing the Source of Medical Distortions

In her book, *The Flight to Objectivity*, Susan Bordo shows how Descartes was pivotal in initiating the mechanistic approach to the body that started the modern scientific movement in medicine. Descartes proposed that neither bodily responses or associated thinking, intuition or emotion can tell us about something; only measurement is an objective tool. Objective medical science transcends the body and allows independence from that body according to Descartes' view. This approach freed doctors from the control of the church and allowed them to study the body as they would any inanimate object.

Descartes' genius is described in his work, *Meditations*: how he translated his experience of estrangement and loss into a vision for the growth of human knowledge and progress.[18] His famous doubt, paired against the ideal of the objectivity which conquered that doubt, appears to be an *unconscious defense against anxiety, or reaction formation, (a neurotic defense)[19]*. Bordo goes on to demonstrate how this highly masculine world view defined by white, upper class males, epitomized by Descartes, became the dominant thinking in our culture affecting everyone until the last sixty years where it has been challenged by, but still clashes with, the more inclusive, feminine view of women, people of color and those from lower and middle class circumstances who are often more in touch with human and cultural wisdom and values. The pursuit of reason or objectivity is seen as a masculine defense in that it gives the illusion of certainty in a multi-dimensional world where many factors do not lend themselves to statistical analysis. The feminine view is seen as more in touch with the body, the rhythms of life and death, and the role of emotion and intuition in the healing process.

This pursuit of objectivity as a defense has affected our whole society; but particularly the medical profession today. As modern-day doctors have become more anxious about lawsuits and their livelihoods,

[18] Susan R. Bordo, *The Flight to Objectivity: Essays on Cartesianism and Culture*, SUNY Series in Philosophy (New York: State University of New York, 1987).p 100
[19] See George E Vaillant, *The Wisdom of the Ego,* (Harvard University Press, 1993) p65

they have become more and more focused on technology as a way to wrest certainty from the medical encounter. But since emotion and intuition affect everything in the medical world including what gets studied by medical scientists and the types of medications offered by the pharmaceutical companies, and since the meaning of any symptom determines when a patient seeks out medical help, a purely technical approach can be very limiting.

Even the very objective (biological rather than psychological) direction that psychiatry has taken in its professional focus and diagnostic systems in recent years can be seen in part as a reaction to anxiety over the inroads psychologists, other counselors, and even psychiatric nurses have made into the psychiatric marketplace. Even so, awareness of defense mechanisms and how they affect everyone has penetrated the culture and crept back into the diagnostic manual that mental health professionals use.

CHAPTER TEN

UNDERSTANDING CULTURAL ILLUSIONS

A physician is obligated to consider more than a dis-
eased organ, more even than a whole man—he must
view the man in his world.
—Harvey Cushing, MD

The second factor I found that accounted for the difference in policy positions people took, had to do with cultural illusions or beliefs people pick up from their culture. Anthropologists Margaret Mead and Ernest Becker helped me understand how different policy makers (or groups of physicians or others) can adopt different sets of such seemingly inconsistent beliefs. Mead studied children in the Samoan Islands to see whether they believed in animism, the religion of the islanders, more than American children who were not exposed to the ideas. She found neither children in the United States nor in the Samoan Islands believed in animism;[20] It took fifteen years of exposure to animism for the Samoan children to accept their culture's religion.

Ernest Becker, on the other hand, surveyed known information about human beings and noted that although humans have the capacity to see what is happening beyond their own circumstances, they have difficulty seeing what is going on immediately around them.[21] This blindness

---

[20] Margaret Mead, *Coming of Age in Samoa* (New York: Perennial Classics Edition, Harper Collins,1928).

[21] Ernest Becker, *The Birth and Death of Meaning* (New York: Free Press, 1971).

comes from years of education and training by families, communities, religious groups, schools, books, television, and even professions. Every generation is indoctrinated into its own set of beliefs, which blinds them somewhat to aspects of reality that might be obvious to someone from a different background or culture. This teaching imparts lessons important to survival in that particular culture, but it may blind a person to ideas outside their cultural norm and contributes to prejudices and biases that are always present if not always conscious.

No matter how hard we work at being objective by peeling away the layers of indoctrination from our families, communities, religious groups, the media, and our professions, we are all affected by subtle and not-so-subtle biases that structure our world. On the positive side, such teachings help us to survive, to deal with anxiety, and to participate as members of a larger social group. These life lessons even teach us how to manage pain most of the time, but they also make it harder to see things from another's point of view.

Every generation can see the ignorance and errors of the generation before, but it cannot see its own. In 1847, before the discovery that germs cause illness, Ignác Semmelweis, the Hungarian physician who was called the "savior of mothers" for his discovery that hand washing decreased the incidence of childbed fever, was run out of town in disgrace when he suggested that physicians were causing childbed fever by bringing contaminants on their hands from the morgue. It was only after his death that the discovery of germs by Dr. Louis Pasteur vindicated Semmelweis and his views became accepted. This story was only one treasure I found in Eugene Robins's book, *Matters of Life and Death: The Risks and Benefits of Medical Care*,[22] which traces the history of humanity's folly in the medical profession. Robins explains how belief in the traditional and prescribed, *rather than observation of the patient* and what is actually going on, affects what doctors do and how they treat their patients.

---

[22] Eugene D. Robin, *Matters of Life and Death: Risks vs. Benefits of Medical Care* (Stanford, CA: Stanford University Press, 1984).

Cultural Illusion: The Belief in Scientific Medicine

In medicine, astonishing advances in science and technology have fueled the illusion of certainty in an uncertain medical world. But unlike plate tectonics or particle physics, medicine deals with human beings. So how can scientific medicine, a purely statistical method, take into account a patient's needs, purpose or motivation, all of which are important to health and healing. In America we have so worshiped the scientific method that sweeping changes in behavior have followed a single scientific study of health activity or diet.

The stunning advances in geology, physics and even medical technology overshadow the very human issues that must be addressed by medicine. Even government action which regulates all those activities that promote health or human destruction, must respond to human needs and human values. At times the whole society has become so enslaved by statistics we forget that numbers do not create anything, especially values and meaning.

Culture, not science, teaches about diet, relationships, the good and the bad, and how to take care of ourselves and stay healthy. American medical culture instead has brought us the medical model and an attempt to dehumanize the process of healing.

An Expert Confronts the Limitations of Science

At a 1980s psychiatric meeting in Chicago, I heard Dr. John Davis, a well-known psycho-pharmacologist, present his work. In the question-and-answer period, someone pointed out, "Dr. Davis, your data doesn't fit the theory."

To his credit, Davis laughed and, in a moment of candor, told this story: "When I was in training," he said (more or less as I remember it), "I was so glad not to be going into psychoanalysis, which appeared to me to be just a lot of guesswork. I was glad I was dealing with hard science, something one could depend on. Now I see that science operates just like psychoanalysis! We just call our guesswork *theory*. Sometimes the theory's right, and sometimes it's wrong!"

I appreciated his candor. All advances in our knowledge are made in part by intuition or guesswork, and in part by experimentation or experience. Even in physics, the history of advancement is of this kind: some by intuition and some by experimentation. It is true of medicine as well. And, it means that some experiments fail and some intuition is wrong, but it also means that slavish reliance on technology and medications may severely limit what physicians have to offer those in desperate need of intervention.

CHAPTER ELEVEN

PLACEBOS AND NOCEBOS

*Some patients though conscious that their condition is
perilous, recover their health simply through their con-
tentment with the goodness of the physician.*
—Hippocrates

The Placebo Effect: Getting the Story Right

It has always been a bit of a mystery to me why doctors had such
trouble with the placebo effect and the role of belief in medical treatment. It has always seemed to me the most rational part of the whole
healing ritual. Ah, the power of belief! Doctors see it routinely in the
placebo effect and still mistrust it. Yet this placebo effect, a belief in the
cure, is the crux of the healing role physicians play. Doctors have been
so convinced that any improvement attributable to the placebo effect is
just trickery that they tend to discount the lessons of the placebo effect
throughout history.

Part of the problem lies with our association of placebos with the
placebo trial in medical research. Here dummy pills are compared to
the drug we want to evaluate for efficacy. Both patients and doctors
are blind to which substance is the dummy pill and which is the real
medicine. But placeboes are more complicated than that. Placebos
have nothing to do with deception or lying. They have to do with
finding a story or an activity that the patient can relate to that helps
him or her live with the reality of what is happening. Humans are

symbolic beings. They live with symbolic constructs that help them master particular tasks. When we are sick we go to the doctor who gives us a pill to make us well. The pill may have no effect on our particular problem, but our belief in the healing power of that pill starts the healing process. The question is not about truth or reality; it is about survival and finding constructs that facilitate healing that do not lead to depression or a sense of hopelessness and despair which can make us worse.

The polar opposite of the placebo is the *nocebo*. Nocebos are stories we believe that make us ill (or more ill) or even kill us. A nocebo causes an adverse reaction due to a belief that a situation, substance, or treatment will bring harm—whether it is capable of doing so or not. A voodoo curse that brings about death once it has been placed on someone is an example of a nocebo. All manner of negative beliefs can keep individuals from getting better. Doctors need to be sensitive to the deleterious effects of any negative information or behavior that may act as a nocebo and be ready to intervene when a patient's progress is delayed by that negative event or belief.

Understanding the Placebo Effect

The history of medical treatment has been described as the history of the placebo effect, which means that much of the benefit of medical treatment is due to a patient's belief in what the doctor is doing.[23] Physicians try to control the intrusion of placebos into the world of scientific medicine, but the placebo effect takes place in spite of what a doctor thinks he or she is doing. The more a doctor believes in the efficacy of medicine, the more beneficial it is likely to be. The placebo effect is enhanced by suggestion, so doctors who dismiss it as quackery may fail to take advantage of this benefit to their patients.

The notion of the placebo came about when doctors substituted dummy pills to keep their patients happy. If the patient wanted a pill the

---

[23] Heiner Fruehauf, "Science, Politics and the Making of TCM," *Journal of Chinese Medicine* 61 (October 1999): 3.

doctor did not think would help, or might be addicting, then the patient would be placated with sugar pills. This was especially true of pain medicine, nerve pills, and sleeping medicine. Only gradually did doctors realize that all medicines and medical treatments had some placebo effect. Now, to determine whether the effects of a new drug are *real* or are *just a* placebo effect, a test group is given the new substance or procedure while a control group is given an inert version—neither group nor the treating physician knows which version they have received—and the effects are compared.

Even diagnostic tests may have some placebo effect. One of my patients thanked me for ordering an electrocardiogram (EKG) heart test for her and told me how much better she felt after the test! In this day of scientific medicine, physicians believe so strongly in pills and surgeries that they convince patients to believe in the treatments as well. Belief and suggestion reinforce the placebo effect. Certainly, the pharmaceutical industry banks heavily on patients' belief in pills, and it spends huge amounts of money advertising and lobbying to promote such belief. Even knowing this, many physicians discount any potential benefits of the placebo effect.

Understanding the Placebo Effect Has Been Slow

Not only has the placebo effect challenged the scientist's search for objective reality, but understanding the placebo effect has only come about in stages . The *Oxford English Dictionary* defines *placebo* as "medicine given to humor, rather than cure, the patient; a dummy pill."[24] But that so-called dummy pill has turned out to be very powerful medicine and not easy to replicate. That's because placebos appear to be responses to a strong belief that causes the release of endorphins. We know this because placebo effects can be blocked by narcotic antagonists—medicines that block the effect of drugs on the opiate receptors in the brain and thus also of opiates in the body. Narcotic antagonists do not affect conditioned

---

[24] Anne Harrington, *The Placebo Effect: An Interdisciplinary Explanation* (University Press, 1999), 13.

responses,[25] hypnosis or relaxation responses. These affect other neuro-chemicals and other parts of the brain.

Homeopathy (a system of alternative medicine that Samuel Hahnemann originated in 1796) was discounted by modern medicine until its potential for creating placebo responses was demonstrated. Even surgical procedures produce a placebo effect. This has been demonstrated in cases where surgery was stopped after an incision but before the procedure was completed. In one placebo/surgery trial, some patients had lasting cures with only a skin incision.

Placebos Must Not be Confused with Conditioned Responses

That so-called dummy pill given after a patient has been taking an opi-ate for pain turns out not to generate a placebo response, at all. It causes a *conditioned response*—much like that of Pavlov's dogs. By ringing a bell every time he presented the dogs with food, Pavlov trained his dogs to salivate at the sound. Giving a shot or a pill to relieve pain, conditions the patient to respond to a pill or a shot.

Even animals can be conditioned to some effects of a drug, which can then be continued by giving a sugar pill. Of course, the animals do not know what the drug was being given for in the first place. That means that events that change the nervous system, like those caused by opiate use, can be reinforced by associated events or even objects like needles or pills. In medicine, we doctors have to be sure that our associ-ated activities reinforce the good results we want, not unwanted effects. Placebo responses are different from conditioned responses.

Doctors Have Difficulty with the Placebo Concept

The difficulty physicians have with the placebo concept was brought home to me while I served on the medical advisory board of the Mul-tiple Sclerosis Society. We were reviewing articles submitted for publi-

---

[25] Harrington, *The Cure Within*, 133.

cation in the MS newsletter. At one meeting in the early 1990s, an article on the effectiveness of physical exercise was submitted to the board. The consensus was against publishing it, because exercise had not been proven scientifically to be of benefit in multiple sclerosis.

"It's probably just a placebo effect," said one of the physicians, discounting the article. His point was that it was not the exercise itself that made the difference, but the fact that the patient believed it did.

I spoke up. "The history of medical treatment has been said to be the history of the placebo effect."

"Yes, that's true," said one of the neurologists. "Even interferon… the big treatment for multiple sclerosis… has some placebo effect."

The other physicians looked at him in amazement. "It does?" they asked. They had all come to believe that at least this treatment for multiple sclerosis was different.

That is not to say that medicines or surgery do not have effects other than placebo effects, but the healing of the body comes from within, and it is too easy to forget the influence of the placebo effect, to believe completely in a new really effective drug, and ignore the fact that belief ensures its positive effect—but it is exactly that kind of conviction that persuades patients to take drugs in the first place, and to believe they will be helped.

Recent studies have confirmed that endorphins, painkillers that occur naturally in different parts of our brains, are the source of the benefit we call the placebo effect.[26] This is not new information; we have known for at least twenty-five years that the placebo effect can be blocked by narcotic antagonists like naloxone. The puzzle is why doctors are still skeptical about the placebo effect. I think the reason is twofold. In the search for dependable facts, that is, real medicine and real treatments, doctors do not really understand what the placebo effect is or how it fits into modern day practice. Doctors just are not trained in how to make placebos work to help their patients. The

---

[26] Jon-Kar Zubieta et al., "Placebo Effects Mediated by Endogenous Opioid Activity on μ-opioid Receptors," *Journal of Neuroscience* 25, no. 34 (August 2005): 7754–7762.

paradox is this: our own nervous system contains the mechanisms for removing the pain it produces, as well as the mechanisms for healing and getting well, but it also has the capacity to make us hurt, give up, and die. The doctor's role in this involves more than a pill, but it takes a mindset that is different from the current medical model. Here is an example.

One day, I was asked to see two men in their forties who had recently been diagnosed with acute leukemia, a fatal disease. One man was smiling. He was surrounded by family and members of his church and saying, "God must have brought me this test for a reason. He must have a purpose for my life, even though I don't know what that is right now."

The other man was lying in bed alone, the sheet over his head, hardly talking. "What is there to talk about?" he said when I pressed him. "The doctors tell me the leukemia is fatal." Though their blood work looked identical, the second man died in a matter of days, while the first man lived months longer than expected by his physicians. What we believe about our lives and circumstances are powerful forces that direct our behavior through tough times. We all have to die today or tomorrow, but how we live and how we die are at least as important as the number of days, and this is where physicians can make a difference if they see caring for their patients as more than presenting facts or treating the numbers on the chart with another chemical.

The Eye Can See, Even If It Does Not Know How

As Loren Eiseley so wisely observed, "You don't have to know how the eye works in order to see."[27] In the same way, we can heal ourselves and be relieved of pain without knowing how we did it. This does not depend on weak-mindedness; it depends on trusting the wisdom of the body to heal itself in ways we are only beginning to understand. Healing can occur in response to love, a kiss, a touch, a belief in God, a pill in the hand of a wise healer—anything. But the physician has to be sure he

---

[27] Loren Eiseley, *The Star Thrower* (New York: Random House, 1979).

does not blunder in and make things worse. There are times we all are vulnerable and need support to do better.

And it does not even matter if what we believe is true!

Not Everyone Is a Placebo Responder

One reason the placebo concept has been hard for doctors to accept is that people are not all the same. It appears that only one person in three is a placebo responder. The number can be increased by another third with suggestion—a reinforcing, positive message that makes the person respond. Yet, belief or suggestion do not awaken the response for everyone, just as some people have musical ability and others do not, and some are hypnotizable and others are not.

Another reason placebo effects have been difficult for physicians to accept is that we have an incomplete understanding of how the brain works—along with some confusion about truth and reality! There is a difference between beliefs that we accept as true and facts as they actually exist, but most of the time facts are confounded by multiple factors and the search for reality a mere illusion.

Reason and Mythology

Before the time of Isaac Newton in the seventeenth century, Westerners accepted the dual realms of reason and mythology.[28] Reason encompassed what was rational, logical, and knowable. It was the practical means for solving problems and functioning well in the world. Mythology had to do with values and giving meaning to things that could not be plainly seen or rationally explained. Mythology connected people to their cultures, their history, and one another. And mythology gave meaning to existence by connecting man to the eternal and the universal.

We sometimes fail to recognize that reason alone cannot assuage all human pain or suffering, deal with sorrow, or give meaning to

---

[28] Karen Armstrong, *A History of God* (New York: Ballantine Books, 1993).

tragedy. Our collective stories, like those in the Bible, Koran, and even Shakespeare, address the meaning and value of human life.

Pain and Getting the *Right Story*

Nowhere is mythology or having the right story more important than in the treatment of pain. Recovery from chronic pain means sufferers must do something different: change how they move, what they eat, how they spend the day. Doctors cannot just heap on more pills to eliminate the pain; they have to provide a story that encourages patients to do what they need to do to get better day by day.

Human beings operate a lot like servomechanisms. That is, if they have a goal, they try different strategies until they reach their goal. It is said that those who succeed in life fail more often than those who fail: because when one strategy does not work, they try something else until they get the job done. If people do not set goals or expect something of themselves, nothing changes. That is where myth, or the medical story, becomes important. The physician's vision must include all the factors that contribute to the pain,[29] not just the diagnosis. Then the physician must embrace a scenario where goal setting, practice, reevaluation, and new goal setting move the patient toward the desired outcome.

In this day of stunning high-tech successes in medicine and surgery, we sometimes forget about the wisdom of the body and the power of the mind—the body's capacity to manage the pain it creates and to bring about healing, and the patient's will to live or to give up and die. These factors make a difference.

As a young doctor, I heard about the man who broke the five-minute mile after his doctors told him he would never walk again. What gives someone the determination to overcome difficulty? Why do others give in and give up? Obviously, there are many factors. The runner's determination not to be limited by a doctor's predictions (which were based

---

[29] Factors contributing to pain include medical causes, damaged nerves, tight muscles and tendons, emotional factors like depression, anxiety, anger, stress, inactivity, lack of interest in activities, social withdrawal, and negative thinking.

only upon statistical probability, anyway) made the difference. Maybe 95 percent of similar patients never do walk again. But while science must look at probabilities, those practicing medicine must make sure that negative messages—nocebos—do not lead the patient to be one of the 95 percent instead of one of the 5 percent. For patients, a doctor's belief in them and in their capacity to overcome what faces them needs to be part of the mythology of medicine. Without it, what doctors have to offer patients with chronic pain, depression, and other chronic conditions can make them worse.

Giving Bad News: Avoiding Medical Nocebos

Doctors have debated throughout the twentieth century how much to tell patients about their conditions: enough so that they can be prepared and take appropriate action, but not so much that they just give up and die. Doctors sometimes forget that other information can be as devastating as a death sentence. Hearing the doctor say, "You're always going to hurt! You'll just have to live with it!" can signal the end of life, just like, "There is nothing more that can be done." Statements like that have always infuriated me because they only mean that *this* doctor has reached the end of his or her own capacity to deal with the situation. Even when someone is dying, there is always more that can be done, if only to ease the pain and suffering (anxiety, depression and sleeplessness,) and be there with the patient at the end. Saying nothing can be done not only robs the patient of a chance to grieve with someone who cares about his or her plight, but makes it sound like the quality of the life that remains is a secondary consideration. The worst thing about dying or being chronically ill is not that you have to die or that you become incapacitated; it is what being sick does to relationships. People back off. There are the ritualized and obligatory contacts, but too often, the warmth and intimacy of being alive slips away before the music has stopped.

Some doctors think that forcing patients to accept harsh realities from the outset can be beneficial, so they tend to give the harshest news and the worst diagnosis, even when they may be wrong! But doctors are safer if they structure a positive message rather than a discouraging and hopeless one. This is especially true if they have nothing of substance to offer.

During the course of having multiple sclerosis, I experienced a lack of connection with a caring physician several times. When I was fifty-five, a new treatment came out for multiple sclerosis: (beta) interferon. I thought I should see an expert in multiple sclerosis about taking the drug. When I called the neurologist I had been working with for some time, he said, "Send me your latest MRI results."

"I've never had one," I replied.

"You've never had an MRI?" he asked, amazed.

I said, "I didn't see any point. What was it going to tell me that I didn't already know?"

When I went to see him, I gave him my history of my symptoms. He asked, "You've never been hospitalized or had cortisone for an episode, either?" He sounded amazed that I had not sought medical attention for every episode.

"I didn't see any point in going when I couldn't see that it would do me any good. I might not have been able to read some times, or had to hold on to the wall some days, but I never missed a day's work," I told him.

He sent me for two MRIs and some evoked potential tests. These confirmed the diagnosis of multiple sclerosis and the damage I had described to him. When I went back to get the results, he told me, "You're not eligible for interferon, because you have chronic progressive MS." I knew that was the worst kind.

I looked at him in disbelief and was suddenly filled with rage at the stupidity of the medical system. What he should have said was, *You're lucky! You don't need to take the treatments, because you haven't had any new symptoms for a while.* Or even, *Your MS might be arrested, since you haven't had any new symptoms for some time.* But even if he did not want to go that far, he could have made me feel good about how I was doing instead of telling me I had the worst kind of multiple sclerosis and was not eligible for his medicine! Giving me a terrible diagnosis may have made him feel he was doing his job, but it left me feeling not only fearful about the future, but like the worst kind of pariah: someone no one was interested in helping anymore! Why, he did not even need to run all those expensive tests that told me not one thing I did not already know in order to tell me I was not eligible for his study! Of course he would not want me for his study, because I had not had a new symptom for years! So how could he tell if the medicine was doing anything? Whatever happened to "Do no harm"? And I remember thinking, *And he didn't even question me closely to see what I might be doing right!*

Even though the new treatment, interferon, made patients sick for twenty-four to forty-eight hours every week, my own patients just starting out with multiple sclerosis who went on interferon, instantly felt better because they were not afraid of what the multiple sclerosis would do to them next. Whether interferon would do what it promised was still being studied then, but it was a boon to those living with the sword of Damocles over their heads. My neurologist visit confirmed to me the importance of approaching patients with a positive story, especially when you have nothing to offer! It also taught me the importance of anger in a world that is not always caring and just. Fortunately, I was able to channel the energy in that anger into writing this book and rejoice in the fact that I did not have to be a patient for the rest of my life.

FINDING
THE
PATH
TO
RECOVERY

CHAPTER TWELVE

LESSONS FROM THE POOR: COPING WITH DEPRESSION AND PAIN

It's very expensive to give bad medical care to poor people in a rich country.
—Paul Farmer, MD

As a psychiatrist, I divided my practice between treating hospital patients with severe mental illnesses, treating outpatients with medication, and individual, family, or group psychotherapy in my office. I had always had a special interest in working with medical patients and in teaching medical students about the things psychiatrists understand best, so when my children were grown, I looked for ways to shift what I was doing. I thought about returning to research and getting a degree in international public health. I even visited the World Health Organization in Geneva to assess job possibilities. The year was 1989.

As part of my search, I talked with an old friend, Dr. Max Michael. We had worked together with Healthcare for the Homeless, and I wanted to see if there might be some way to be more involved with his activities. Max was the head of medicine at Cooper Green Hospital, the local county hospital for the poor and uninsured.

He came to my house one blustery Sunday afternoon. As we sat in front of the fire with warming drinks in our hands, he said, "You know, don't you, that your profession is bankrupt." He paused to see if I was with him. "The people psychiatry was meant to help are out there wandering the streets, homeless, without access to the psychiatric system.

The mentally ill who should be locked up in a hospital for safety, are often in jail, without access to proper treatment and care." I could see him relive his struggles to get help for the homeless mentally ill he treated every day. He went on, "And psychiatric education isn't much better. Our medical students are graduating and becoming doctors without being able to recognize garden variety anxiety and depression in their patients.

"Would you be willing to teach medical students and young doctors on the medical wards—where the action really is? And would you take on medical patients with psychiatric problems that other physicians in the hospital or clinics would like you to see?" He paused. "You could do case presentations in morning report every other week, and use these patients to teach young doctors and medical students what they need to know." He was thinking it out as he spoke.

A job like that presented the opportunity of a lifetime for me. For years, I had been teaching medical students about anxiety, depression and pain, and addiction through lectures in pharmacology and then medicine. At Cooper Green, I could use my knowledge to help patients with a variety of medical problems, and educate medical students and young doctors at the same time. Max suggested that I start in three months. I would work one day a week, and we would grow from there. I was thrilled. Little did I know then what challenges lay ahead, or what it would take to see it through.

A Short History of Cooper Green Hospital

I came to Alabama at the height of the civil rights activities in 1964, to take a medical internship with Dr. Tinsley Harrison. I remember the Friday nights when the old Hillman emergency room filled with victims from the poor communities who had been in fights: knife fights, gun battles, bar fights, domestic rows. It was a weekly event. Eventually, the county built Cooper Green hospital five blocks down the road to treat the indigent population. Cooper Green hired its own doctors, but the faculty and medical students from the University rotated through all the services. By 1990, Cooper Green housed two nationally famous programs: the AIDS treatment program known as the Saint George's Clinic, and the end-of-life program known as the Balm of Gilead. Cooper Green was always short of money, but it had the support and enthusiasm of the wider community.

Many of the patients who come to Cooper Green live in neighborhoods where violence and theft is a part of daily life. Most have little or no money. Even those on disability, welfare, or social security have little to support all their needs. There is no reliable public transportation, so they are dependent on those who can give them a lift to get to work. Most have lost family members and friends to violence, illness, or incarceration. Of those coming to Cooper Green, the most responsible take care of sick family members and children whose parents are in jail or have to work. Many have children and grandchildren who have only known one parent and grieve that their fathers never acknowledged them. They may have witnessed parents or spouses blow their brains out; been exposed to drugs, alcohol, or other violence at an early age; or been in jail themselves. Selling drugs or their own prescriptions is commonplace. Some would not have a place to live or food in their mouths if they did not sell their medicines.

Many patients are African-American, but there are many whites who come to Cooper Green as well. Cooper Green serves the uninsured as well as the poor. The clinic itself is staffed by an ethnically and internationally diverse group of doctors, medical assistants, and physical therapists. Most of the nurses are African-American from the local community.

My First Day at Cooper Green

The first day I went to Cooper Green, Max showed me around the medical clinic and introduced me to the staff. Our first stop was an office at one end of the clinic, where the head nurse sat behind her desk. "Dr. Carmichael will be seeing patients with depression in the clinic every Friday," he told her after making introductions. "Any thoughts about where I should put her?"

"We don't have anything but the small conference room," she said, clearly annoyed at not knowing of my arrival ahead of time. "We don't get coffee or other things for the doctors around here," she asserted, looking at my cane. "You're expected to get things for yourself." Since I had been a medical student at Bellevue Hospital, the public hospital in New York City, I fully expected to have to pitch in. But her surliness was noted.

Next, I was taken to meet the clerks in the front office. These women checked in patients and would let me know when someone was there to see me. They sat behind a large window facing a line of sick people waiting to check in. Some patients looked so frail I wanted to rush out and find them a chair, but even though this waiting room was a fair size, there were no chairs to be seen. As I went to see my first patient, I made a mental note that courtesy and kindness were not a high priority in this clinic.

The tiny conference room I had been assigned was in the middle of the medical clinic itself. The room had a small table and two or three old plastic chairs. Remnants of someone's snack from the day before and an array of papers of one kind or another lay on the table. Two darkened X-ray boxes and a stash of X-rays lying helter-skelter in one corner lent silent testimony to the multiple uses of this tiny space. As I cleared the remnants of the food, wiped the table, and stacked the papers and X-rays so they were not so distracting, I was introduced to my first patient.

The woman who was ushered into my room was tall and gaunt and slightly bent at the shoulders, like someone holding up the weight of the world. I did not have to ask her to tell me her symptoms to see that she was depressed. She pulled a tissue out, and I introduced myself and told her what I was doing in the clinic.

"My name is Mattie Harris," she introduced herself. "My only son was killed in Iraq, and I can't seem to get over it." A tear escaped the tissue she was holding to her eyes and nose and rolled down her cheek. "He enlisted in the marines when he was only eighteen years old to make something of himself," she said in barely a whisper. "We were all so proud." In the hall, I could hear a nurse calling for someone as the patient gathered herself. "We got the telegram Christmas week."

"I can't imagine anything worse," I said, trying to imagine what it would be like to lose my son like that.

More tears followed as this quiet woman went on gradually with her story. "I take care of my parents and my grandmother. They're old and sick. I don't think they will last much longer. My son was trying to help with some money each month, but things have been very tight since he died, and I'm afraid that soon I won't be able to do everything they need. My back has been bothering me more and more, and the pills they give me don't seem to do much good anymore."

I asked questions about her depression, pain, sleep, appetite, and day-to-day activities. "Have you been to physical therapy?" I finally inquired.

"The doctors sent me last year," she answered after a pause, "but it was expensive and it made me worse, so I stopped going. Now I have trouble doing much of anything."

"What have the doctors told you to do about your back?"

"Just to take the pills if it hurts too much, but they are too expensive to take very often."

As I listened to this woman, I felt increasingly angry with a system that does not help patients like this get better. In spite of being a doctor, I had had similar trouble getting the help I needed with my own physical problems. Even for me, the medicines were too expensive to keep taking and did not really solve anything. I began telling Mrs. Harris my own story of recovery from chronic pain. She stopped crying and listened intently to every word.

"I'm also going to give you some medicine for the depression," I said. "It should help with some of your symptoms, and I will be able to give you free samples. Still, the most important thing you can do for yourself is to walk and stretch every day, preferably with a friend, so you can take a break and have some support. I want to see you in two weeks so we can talk some more and I can see how you are doing with the walking and the medicine."

She walked out of the room standing taller and thanked me for my help. Little did I suspect that it would be a year before I saw her again.

When she did come back, she looked like a different woman. "You don't remember me," she said, noting my confusion as I looked at her chart and then at her. "I'm not surprised." She was smiling and eager to talk. She was right; I didn't immediately recognize her. It had been a long time, and she didn't look like the woman I had described in the chart. "You gave me some pills, but it was impossible for me to come back and get more. This is the first chance I've had to come since I saw you last. My grandmother died, and my mother ended up in a nursing home. My niece had to go to work, so I have her two children with me now, but I did what you said about exercise." Listening to her, I could hardly believe this was the same woman I had seen a year before.

She continued, "In the beginning, I was so wobbly that I had to have someone on each side of me when I walked. Now I'm walking two miles a day with a friend, and it's the best part of my life. Thank you."

I was amazed at this woman's determination, especially in the face of so much responsibility and loss. Since then, I have thought many times of Mrs. Harris and how no one had told her about walking or had focused on the importance of doing it daily. I have also mused about the importance of the doctor-patient relationship in bringing about change. "And *it's not time-consuming*!" I want to shout, since there is so much emphasis on being efficient in medicine. I knew that my anger at the plight of Mrs. Harris in the medical system led me to a more empathic response, and this touched her and gave her the tools to make the change.

Most of the patients who came to see me in the clinic had several chronic illnesses, many losses and life stresses, drug or alcohol abuse problems, and very little support or money to do anything about them. Many also had other people to care for along with their own physical and mental problems. A large number of the patients sent to me for depression had chronic pain problems that were being treated only with medications. These patients might have been sent to the physical therapy department at one time or another, but they had no regular exercise or stretching routine and no other interventions to assist them with pain management.

Physical rehabilitation, not just a month of physical therapy aimed at one part of the body, is an essential element in recovery from any chronic illness, but especially when chronic pain is part of the picture. Over the next fifteen years of working with medical patients, I realized what other elements were needed to recover from depression and chronic pain. I would also learn more about how and why modern medical approaches miss the point.

The Power of Courtesy and Respect

Being in the clinic only one half day per week, I was painfully aware of what little I might have to give patients in the short period of time I had with them. So I worked hard not to keep patients waiting. Even from the beginning it was clear that offering this token of respect made a big difference to many of the patients. We forget sometimes the power of courtesy to ease relationships and build community. In a world too often dominated by violence and revenge, a kind word and thoughtful behavior can go a long way. For these patients needing to recover from many losses and injuries, courtesy proved amazingly powerful. Even little tributes helped patients gain self esteem and allowed them to make necessary changes in their behavior. I was shocked to see some of the nurses, themselves one step away from being poor, mistreat patients just because they could. But that was only one of my challenges.

Lessons from Teaching Young Doctors

One morning a week, I went on walking rounds with one of the medical treatment teams, which consisted of a senior attending physician, a medical resident, one or more interns, and several medical students. My job was to comment on patients along the way. The two biggest problem areas I identified were unrecognized suicide attempts and unrecognized delirium or mental confusion from a number of medical causes.

What surprised me the most on rounds was the almost total focus on technology to the exclusion of other observations and information about the patient. This was especially incredible considering that on average, 30 to 40 percent of the patients had behavioral changes due to medical illness or treatment. Even more astonishing was that almost none of the physicians performed a mental status examination on a patient with a behavior change before calling for a psychiatric consult, nor did they speak with the family to find out whether the change in behavior was sudden or just the way the person was all the time.

Mental changes are very common in all medical illnesses because of infection, fever, blood chemistry or oxygen changes, withdrawal from alcohol or drugs, and a whole host of other factors. The medical nature of the change can be identified simply by *asking a few questions and confirming any recent changes with the family.* The causes may be life threatening, but they are treatable—not by the psychiatrist, but by the internist or surgeon. Delay is neither desirable nor necessary.

This disdain for dealing with emotion seemed to be pervasive; even the kindest of physicians seemed oblivious to the patient's mental state. I was truly amazed at the complete lack of interest in a patient's behavior or emotional changes by almost all involved, because these changes are central to the patient's well-being and even survival. One morning on rounds I saw in the nurse's notes that one patient had been talking about the nurses giving her a hard time during the night. The patient appeared clear enough on morning rounds, but when I went back to talk to her I found she was confused about the date and what treatment she was receiving. This patient was suffering from a delirium. She was confused and paranoid in the middle of the night, but apparently clear in the morning, a common pattern. Since delirium must be identified and its cause determined as soon as possible, failure to notice the change at night could harm the patient or someone else should the patient strike out to protect herself in the middle of the night. Talking with family members to determine when a behavior change takes place and realizing the patient may look normal in the morning are important to addressing the problem.

Suicidal behavior was often missed because doctors failed to recognize noncompliant behavior for what it was: heart patients smoking, diabetics failing to take insulin, a patient not showing up for dialysis. Rather than explore the depression and suicidal thoughts behind the behavior, the doctor would renew admonitions to behave and even threaten not to work with the patient if he or she did not comply with requirements. Often, doctors were uncomfortable talking about death or getting their patients to do the same.

One morning on rounds I heard this exchange, "Now if we're going to do by-pass surgery on your heart, you must not smoke any more." As the doctor moved on I heard the patient say, "I don't know that it matters." Later when I went back to talk with the patient, she said to me, " It doesn't matter because I would just as soon row out into the middle of a lake and not come back. My husband died last year and I just haven't cared much since then." Further conversation revealed the patient was depressed.

Another day on rounds we went to see an eighteen-year-old boy who had been diagnosed with juvenile diabetes the year before. He sat silently on the bed looking dejected. "Eddie," the doctor sat on the bed, "You have to take your insulin every day, so it's important not to let yourself run out. You can get a month's supply at a time, so plan ahead. We can have the diabetes nurse come and go through the educational material with you again. Would that would help?" I watched Eddie's face as the doctor spoke. He looked sad and said nothing. After the others left, I sat down by the bed and introduced myself. "I'm Dr. Carmichael. Can you tell me how you happened to run out of medication?" Eddie looked at me and I was not sure he was going to speak. Slowly he turned. "I don't want to take that stuff. Its ruined my life and I've just had enough." Eddie had given up and just stopped taking the insulin. Doctors recognize an overdose of pills as a suicide attempt, but there are many subtle ways patients give up without actively trying to kill themselves.

During one morning report a young doctor related the story of a dialysis patient who had not shown up for dialysis. Her doctor took her to task saying he would not work with her if she did not come in for her regular visits.

"Tell me about your patient's behavior." I said, trying to get at why the patient had not shown up for her appointment.

"This patient was noncompliant," the young doctor answered.

"What does that mean?" I asked.

"It means the patient doesn't do what the doctor says," came the reply.

"I'm not asking what the word *noncompliant* means; I'm asking what is behind the patient's noncompliant behavior. Working with a patient means that you must not only describe behavior; you must also understand the reason for the noncompliance." The young doctor did not know. Patients on dialysis are 400 times more likely to commit suicide than the general population, so recognizing the signs of depression is important to getting the patient into treatment in time. Electric shock therapy may be life saving in these situations.

Failure to recognize the importance of behavior and emotion, from non-compliant behavior to confusion, means the physician cannot act to help the patient at the most critical of times.

CHAPTER THIRTEEN

FINDING THE PATH TO RECOVERY

Natural forces within us are the true healers of disease.
—Hippocrates

In spite of the difficulties with surly nurses, making timely appointments and the resistance of the medical staff to see emotions as anything but an inconvenience, those early days at the county hospital were very rewarding. Almost everything I did, even simple interventions, seemed to make a huge difference to the patients I saw. Many of them thought little of themselves: they lived in a world where most people looked down on them and treated them accordingly. The amazing thing was that once they were directed onto the path toward recovery, they had astounding resources and resilience, overcoming more than I could have imagined. The capacity of many individuals to survive their difficult lives day after day required a strength that was inspiring. Most of us do not want to think that such deprivation and violence exists in our own communities. In these horrendous situations, it seemed like a miracle to be able to give people tools they could use to get some control back in their lives.

Limited as I was by being there only one day a week, I knew these patients needed more than just another pill for depression. I had to see depressed patients frequently, especially in the beginning, to get to know them and understand their problems. Frequent visits are essential to help manage medication, monitor medication side effects, and watch for suicidal thoughts and other self-defeating behaviors. So I set out to see what was possible in that setting.

Group and Community Therapy

What I needed was a system for seeing people every week, so that we met when they needed it—not just when they could get an appointment, which I could not control. I needed regular hours so patients knew when to show up, even if they had not received an appointment card. And I needed a long enough session with each person so I could see what was going on. Lack of transportation was a big problem for so many, and lack of money and other family problems made consistent returns difficult. It was important to have a system that accommodated patients' needs.

Group therapy seemed the ideal solution. I set up two-hour sessions that included an hour and a half of talk therapy and meditation, exercise, or some other teaching at the end. After group, I would see patients on a first-come, first-served basis for medications or individual problems.

The Magic of Group Therapy

It was inspiring to sit in group therapy and watch people with all of life's worst problems—and I mean *all* of them—find simple methods to help themselves and change their lives. These people had a view of life, existence, and even survival that I could only begin to imagine. These were people who had to face death almost daily. They saw illness, poverty, loss, rejection, and abuse every day. The group would give each patient a chance to tell his or her story and an opportunity to support others.

Listening, I wondered, *Do poor people really feel entitled to be taken care of by the government? Or is wanting to be taken care of like wishing for heaven after a hard life? What does it do to a person to feel so hopeless and helpless to do anything about his or her circumstances? I think it's really people like me who feel entitled—entitled to be free of violence and free to make a decent living, get a good education, and raise children in a good environment.* My patients had no such hopes. At the hospital, even among those doing well, losing everything might be just a paycheck away. Even so, individuals found ways to give to others, to make a small difference where they were.

There were many surprises in the groups. In the first place, the group structure was very different from that of private practice. Instead of coming once a week for a specified time, these patients came when they had transportation, were out of medicine, had other reasons to come to the hospital, or were in a crisis. I found myself watching with amazement as patients dealt with suicidal thoughts, early and later traumas, and current frustrations and problems.

Initially, it looked like less than an optimum group setting because the group was different each week. Even so, these patients were able to take the little time they had to talk about what troubled them. Not only were they completely accepting of one another, but they did not seem to have the shame I had so often seen in my private patients. When someone was able to open up about something hard for him or her to admit or talk about, it always opened a door for several others in the group to talk as well. Acknowledging the gift they had given fellow group members encouraged them and others to open up even more. Thus, the group served as a cathartic as well as to encourage or reinforce positive behaviors. Even the size of the group, sometimes up to twenty-four, did not seem to keep patients from accomplishing what they needed to do. I admit I got nervous once the group reached sixteen. I thought I would have to do something fancy like make it into two groups, but no, patients adjusted to any change and helped me make it work.

Dealing with Suicidal Thoughts

One of my early challenges at Cooper Green was that I was seeing a lot of depressed patients who might be suicidal. Since I was there only one day a week, I had to send truly suicidal patients to the mental health center for care. But since almost everyone I saw had suicidal thoughts, and some had even tried to kill themselves, I had to confront the situation. In the end, what I did was to share with them that if they were really suicidal, I needed to get them someplace where they could get the care they needed: "It's not fair to you not to protect you if that is needed, And it's not fair to other group members who come to care about you, for me to try to treat you here if you don't think you can be responsible for your suicidal thoughts by taking yourself to the emergency room, or by letting me know if you're suicidal. If there is any chance you would act on your thoughts we'd better get you to the mental health center where they can keep a closer eye on you." Over and over, patients assured me they would be responsible for their suicidal thoughts and let me know if they were in trouble. If I had any question, I had the family come in and communicated with them in front of the patient.

Several patients I thought might kill themselves surprised me. Susanne McGill was a forty-year-old woman who had used pills to try suicide thirty-nine times. Initially, I wanted to send her to the mental health center, but she agreed not to take pills again if I let her come to group meetings. "Will you promise not to do anything harmful to yourself, either accidentally or on purpose?" I queried. "Only patients who agree can come to group."

"I promise," she said. But each time she came to group, as it began, she said, "I'm taking back my promise."

"What's that all about?" I responded. Then, throwing it open to the group, I would say, "What about the rest of you? Have you thought of hurting yourself this week?"

"My father blew out his brains all over me when I was a child. I can't get the images out of my head even now." Willie Snow spoke up. He had said very little before.

"That happened with my first husband," Patty Norris announced. "I don't think he meant to kill himself, but he was always threatening. I can still see all that blood."

Rose Kane spoke next. "My daughter killed herself when she was twenty-seven." Her voice was shaky as she shared this news. "She'd had a fight with her husband…" Her voice choked. "I've never recovered. She was my baby, and I think of her every day. For a long time, I'd write letters to her as if she could get them. Prayed to God that it had been a mistake and she'd been taken for someone else."

Rhonda Stephens opened up. "I've been suicidal for the past ten years, ever since my husband left me for another woman. We could never have any children, so there's just me." She turned to look at Rose. "But after listening to you and what that was like for you,

I'll never think of suicide again. I wouldn't want to do that to my mother."

These discussions turned out to be beneficial for everyone in the group as they talked about their own thoughts or previous acts, or family suicides. Susanne had to promise not to harm herself before she left group, or else to go to the mental health center.

Only one person ever took an overdose after promising she would not. Norma Stephens came in to group looking very apologetic.
"My boyfriend took me out drinking and then told me he was through. I think I must have been drunk. I just took all the pills I had in my purse. I hope you'll all forgive me for breaking my promise. I'll never do that again. It was just plain stupid." Promises were sacred. Relationships mattered. We all shared a common bond.

Over and over, I was amazed at how well these patients responded to expectations that they could do better. It was almost as if others in their lives did not believe in their strength or did not care. But here in group, people cared, and that made a difference. After group, the waiting time to see me offered more time to talk with people who cared. Everyone was courteous and generous with one another, allowing someone who had an appointment or a bus to catch to the head of the line to see me.

Other Challenges in the Groups

In running the groups, I found that it was important to be genuine and reveal things about myself and my struggles when I sought to encourage, empathize, or exhort, even while I underscored discoveries made by others in the group when I wanted to teach a better way to do things. It was important that they see that I did not think I had all the answers, and that I could see when they had good ideas. It was also important that I recognized their strength and courage in surviving terrible stress and tragedy and their capacity for wisdom in the face of adversity, whatever their educational level or degree of success or failure in life.

Many of the patients did not feel good about themselves because they could no longer work, had little education, and could see no way to move on to something else. My respect for their points of view and wisdom seemed to be important to their recovery from so much loss. One of the real surprises for me was how much wisdom there was in the groups, sometimes from the most unexpected persons. In another setting, these individuals might have been discounted because of their dress, their life stories, or the fact they had received many psychiatric diagnoses.

I loved to tell the group the story of Stuart Margoles, sports reporter for the *Chicago Tribune*, who gave a talk after the election of President George H.W. Bush about the role of the media in politics. He said (more or less): "No politician or reporter would claim to be an intellectual, but they are very fond of quoting intellectuals. The problem is that intellectuals are wrong 50 percent of the time!" He then went on to describe stunning examples of statements made by President Reagan and others that were just simply wrong. He went on, *"It's the people out there in small towns across the country, living quiet lives, who really know what is going on."* He, too, emphasized the strength of those who have survived difficult times.

I also realized that the behavior of these patients, and their symptoms, had to be viewed in context. Defining their behavior as *dysfunctional*, as we do too often in psychiatry, was to pathologize behavior that might have helped patients survive a tough time. In therapy or medicine, it is the doctor's or the therapist's worldview that determines whether a patient's actions are defined as pathological or effective coping. Such values are not set in stone; whether a behavior is labeled as positive or negative depends upon the doctor's cultural standards. Many things contribute to the way we categorize others. I observed patients give encouragement and support to someone when I wanted to take them to task. Working with the group reminded me, as they used to say, "You can't understand another person until you've walked a mile in his shoes." That's when I realized the importance of the group community to all comers.

Knowing I could not have been the first to observe this, I turned to the Internet for information. I discovered the work of Dr. Trigant Burrows. Burrows was one of the original founders of the American Psychoanalytic Association. He began questioning the way psychoanalysis tended to pathologize patients. He discovered that treating groups of patients with similar socioeconomic backgrounds as well as similar problems allowed their own cultural norms to determine what was pathological and what was acceptable. Because of his criticism of psychoanalysis, Burrows was kicked out of the association. (This is another example of the difficulty that people—even doctors—have with criticism.)

All of these experiences reinforced my belief that *suspending judgment and listening to the patient* were important prerequisites to understanding and helping patients from different cultural backgrounds, who thus have different strengths and weaknesses, needs, and possibilities. Doing so reinforces the relationship between the physician and the patient, which is of great importance to the patient who needs encouragement to get better. But it is also important to the physician who spends a lifetime struggling with the care of such patients. But this is especially hard in a culture brought up to believe the view of the dominant white upper class male to the exclusion of all others and to see other cultures, classes, races, genders and even gender orientation as a threat to the status quo.

Regaining Control over Out-of-Control Lives

Since the medications I prescribed for depression need to be taken for weeks or months to have a full effect and many patients were unable to come on a regular basis, I looked for other ways to treat depression while giving patients back some measure of control over their lives.

Two things proved especially powerful to give depressed patients some control: exercise and meditation or stress management techniques. I told patients my story of pain and recovery, and then started them on a daily routine of exercise and also of progressive relaxation. In my private practice, I offered biofeedback and relaxation tapes to my patients, but in the clinic I only had a written handout giving stress management exercises to teach relaxation. I gave it to patients at the initial visit along with admonitions to develop their own exercise and stretching routine. They were encouraged to take what they already knew and fit it into a routine that worked with their schedules. If they could not do much, then they were encouraged to do a little four times a day. The goal was to move every muscle each day and stretch every joint each day.

My own experience with exercise and stretching seemed to serve as a powerful motivator for some. It helped that they could identify with my pain and my difficulties with the medical system. These patients frequently felt that they got second-rate medical care because they were poor, so seeing that all medical care is about the same, even for someone like me, helped.

Because the patients had so little money, I brought medication samples from my private office. The drug companies were very generous, keeping me and the patients supplied. Once more, I noticed the importance of giving things to patients. It was important that this was a personal transaction with me. I even filled out the drug renewal forms for them so that they did not have to make an additional trip to the pharmacy. This token of caring or regard for their comfort seemed to mean a lot, as did my respect for the patients as people.

Happily, while some of their medical care was less than optimum— their long waits to get appointments, long waits to see the doctor in the hospital, long waits in the pharmacy, and an over reliance on pain medication—some of their care was better than that available in private hospitals. Here they had many caring physicians and other health care providers, all kinds of volunteers willing to donate services, and free medicines (even some I myself could not afford to take regularly).

In addition, as we developed services for those in pain, we planned to offer some services that other pain clinics had had to cut because insurance would not cover them. We were able to do this by using volunteer resources, both from among our patients and from the community. For patients, being a volunteer reinforced their own progress while helping someone else, and it enabled them to focus on something outside themselves.

As I watched patients move step-by-step toward getting their lives back, it seemed to me that perhaps the most important aspect of the treatment I provided for them was the care I had for their feelings. I did not see them as just bodies to be mended, but as individuals with unique lives and enormous strengths that could benefit all.

CHAPTER FOURTEEN

THE DEPRESSION-PAIN CONNECTION

All the adversity I've had in my life, all my troubles and
obstacles, have strengthened me......You may not realize
it when it happens, but a kick in the teeth may be the
best thing in the world for you.
—Walt Disney

What Is Depression?

Clinical depression has been recognized since early times, but what causes it has always been debated. Major depressions are known to run in families, as are those that are part of bipolar disorder. Those with a sensitive nervous system, like mine, are prone to develop depression under stress. In addition, certain medical conditions (such as thyroid disease or multiple sclerosis) (See Appendix B) or medication (such as female hormone therapy and blood pressure medications) (See Appendix C) may give rise to depression in anyone. A hard life is more apt to give rise to depression in a culture that expects life to be pain free. But extreme trauma may cause depression in anyone.

Depression itself is more than being unhappy because you failed a test or lost a love. Sleep and appetite may increase or decrease. There is a general loss of interest in life. The world appears hopeless, and one feels helpless to do anything about it. Losing interest often means social withdrawal, lack of activity, or loss of involvement in meaningful work, and ultimately, thoughts of death and/or suicide.

Depression is often accompanied by anxiety and multiple pains: headaches, stomach aches, and all-over muscle aches. (See Appendix D) In its most severe form, depression can cause a person to just vegetate, forgetting to eat or bathe. In these instances, electroconvulsive therapy (ECT) may be lifesaving. For those in a completely vegetative state, those who are severely suicidal, and those with medical conditions that worsen if severe depression is not addressed swiftly, electroconvulsive therapy is still the most effective treatment we have.

Fortunately, many symptoms of depression are treatable with medication. But resolving conflicts, dealing with anger and loss, and finding a way back to full functioning may require the intervention of group, individual, or family therapy to head off self-defeating behavior, negative thinking, or relationship issues. Medication alone is rarely adequate treatment even if an individual appears to be functioning—that is, taking care of day-to-day activities—but functioning is the key to treatment. Where depression leads to negative thinking, a reduction in coping skills, judgment problems, and a decreased ability to perceive, express, and understand emotion, then structured intervention by a trained professional becomes essential.

Depression is defined as a medical condition because it has symptoms, some of which medication can treat. In patients with a variety of medical problems, depression may have multiple causes. Some symptoms can be brought on by the illness itself, but others can be precipitated by trauma, burns, surgery, or medication. Some are brought on by the added stress of serious or chronic illness. Whatever the underlying cause or genetic predisposition, depression involves issues of lifestyle (activity, nutrition and socialization), loss, change of relationships, and emotions like anger and fear. These are human issues and must be dealt with in a human context, not just with pills.

Despite the fact that depression today is seen as a medical problem, many still find it hard to accept that it is not a sign of weakness. Even harder for many to accept is that *depression may even be a necessary step in coming to terms with life*. Every life change brings both a loss and a gain, and all those losses have to be grieved before an individual can go on with the new *reality*.

When I went into psychiatry in the 1970s, one physician said to me, "Psychiatrists are immoral. They pull people away from taking responsibility for their bad moods. They weaken their patients' religious faith." A number of my medical colleagues expressed the same belief in one way or another. They failed to recognize that patients must be encouraged to have faith and to do better step-by-step to recover from depression or from chronic pain. Far from not taking responsibility for their bad moods, they must be encouraged to do just that, one step at a time. Only by reengaging in all aspects of life—physical, emotional, occupational, social, and spiritual—can patients make a full recovery.

Surviving Low Times

Having suffered from depression myself I knew that the worst thing about depression was not feeling like myself. I could remember having trouble talking and withdrawing from everything in my life except what I had to do day to day. My weight was always changing and my sleep was fitful, so I could not always tell I was depressed until I found myself thinking, *People like me shouldn't be born!* Fortunately, I knew I had been a useful person, so those thoughts were evidence that I needed help. Being plagued by negative thoughts could be terrible.

When one is caught up in depression, it seems as if it will never end. Feeling so black is miserable. I remember being at a meeting in Toronto; the spring was beautiful and Prokofiev's *Romeo and Juliet* was inspiring, but I felt so bad that I decided I did not want to live a long time feeling the way I did. But I was lucky. I had children and parents and even patients who needed me, so there was never any question of suicide. Yet, depression invariably made me withdraw from church and other activities, which cut me off from support I could have had. I suppose that is why relationships we cannot get out of serve as the best opportunity for using mature defenses. *You have to stick in there, even when the going gets tough: keep going even when you don't feel like it.* My obligations to parents, children, and patients sustained me through many years.

Somewhere along my way, I read about Abraham Lincoln's depressions. A man who had suffered many early losses and disappointments, Lincoln handled his depressions (which reached psychotic proportions on at least one occasion) with humor and a drive to make a difference for others.[30] How was I so blessed to be in a position to make a difference to others rather than end my life? Was it the early training in my family to soldier on in spite of difficulty? Was it the inspiration of the Christian message to love and give to others? Was it the sense of obligation to children, parents, and patients? Was it the realization that I was only truly free of my own misery if I focused on the needs of others? Or parts of all of these?

Hand in Hand with Chronic Pain

When I went to Cooper Green, I expected to see patients with depression, but I was totally unprepared to find the number of depressed patients suffering with chronic pain, especially pain that was being addressed exclusively with opiates. I knew that everyone with chronic pain had to be evaluated for depression, whatever the cause of the pain, because depression is so common—but I had not realized just how common. Chronic pain is more than the aches and pains we manage year after year from wear and tear on our joints or even the aches and pains from old injuries. Chronic pain involves a change where one's whole life centers around managing discomfort and suffering. Statistics show that two out of three people who suffer with chronic pain are *depressed, discouraged, and inactive.*

Depression alone can give rise to a variety of painful conditions. How much this pain results from the effects of the depression—that is, social withdrawal, lack of interest in much of anything, and inactivity—and how much is the direct result of the depression may be hard to tell, but often the two go hand in hand. At least one of Dr. Kevorkian's

---

[30] Joshua Wolf Shenk, *Lincoln's Melancholy: How Depression Challenged a President and Fueled His Greatness* (New York: Houghton Mifflin,1906).

assisted-suicide patients, one who wanted to die because of intolerable pain, showed no evidence of any physical cause for the pain at autopsy.

Treatment, then, involves *reversing the destructive consequences of inactivity, social withdrawal, and lack of meaningful work.* Anyone with chronic pain should be evaluated for depression, and the depression should be treated with medication and talk therapy for the duration of the chronic pain. Talk therapy, psychotherapy, counseling—whatever it is called—sets up a situation that allows for maturation of defense mechanisms over time, resulting in less self-defeating behavior and better coping mechanisms. Such a shift may be essential to full recovery. Those with more debilitating depressions may need the structure of activity and occupational therapy as well.

Two patients underscored for me the role of depression in those with chronic pain. One day, I was asked to see a hospitalized patient who had depression. Mrs. Susan Groves had been in a motorcycle accident four years before, and all she could do was complain about how much pain she had. This was in the early 1990s when doctors were still uncomfortable using opiates to treat chronic pain unless the patient was dying.

I could see as I entered the room that she looked depressed. "Of course I'm depressed," she said defiantly. "What do you expect with a jerk of a husband who hides all the money so I can't get my fair share? I'd probably have killed myself, but I'm not going to give that two-timer the satisfaction of having me out of his life!"

She hurt too much to be very active, so she sat and watched television most of the day. Because it hurt too much to cook, she ordered take-out meals and had gained a considerable amount of weight. She had difficulty sleeping because it was hard to find a comfortable position at night, and she had lost interest in most of her hobbies, though she was a bright and talented woman. Her doctors were baffled, because her injuries had healed well; they thought she should be doing better.

Another patient, Mrs. Evelyn Woods, was sent to me in the clinic to be treated for depression. She had not had any injury or surgery, but she had gained weight with each of her four pregnancies and was more than one hundred pounds overweight. She now had type 2 diabetes. She took pills for it but found it hard to follow the food plan because she had so much stress at home. "My husband's in jail for selling crack cocaine," she told me. "The children help with money, but I know they resent it. I've got my husband's mother living with me. She's got Alzheimer's, so I can't do too much. I guess I just sit around, watch TV, and eat."

Mrs. Woods had pains in all her joints, but her back bothered her the most. The doctors looked at X-rays of her back but did not think she had enough arthritis to explain the amount of pain she had. She also complained of headaches and stomach aches, but nothing was found after an MRI of her head and an X-ray of her colon. This woman, like Susan Groves, was overwhelmed, depressed, and inactive.

In both cases, the treatment amounted to getting the patient going again. For Mrs. Woods, this meant first getting her to talk out her anger while beginning medications for pain and depression. Then she was encouraged to begin the exercises she was able to do, to join a group of others in her situation to get support and encouragement for the changes she was making, and finally, to find a part-time job to both bring in some money and get her out of the house.

The chronic pain problems of these two patients were complicated by depression and difficult life situations. More than medicine for pain and depression, their treatment involved getting them moving again, dealing with their feelings, and encouraging them to be less isolated. Weight issues related to inactivity and the modern American fast food diet we addressed in our patient led groups.

Pain and Denial

Pain is sometimes the way depression expresses itself for people in denial about being depressed. I have seen this most often in ministers and others very involved with religious activity. These people see their depression as a lack of faith in God and, as such, unacceptable. For these patients to see their depression as a medical problem that can be treated with medication, not as a sign of weakness, can be very help-ful. Recognizing the problem and treating the patient's depression with medication and exercise can save the patient a lot of grief. Even though these patients may resist looking at areas of their lives that contribute to the depression, they may be more available to work on their underlying conflicts as their depression responds to medication.

Any illness may be affected by life stresses and the presence of depression and must be addressed if the individual is to return to full functioning. But their role of depression and stress in the production and maintenance of pain has been more difficult to define. Such confusion often leads to a failure to address aspects of rehabilitation that have to do with feelings, relationships, occupation, and security.

Depressed, Discouraged, and Inactive

Understanding the depression-pain connection can help correct stereotypes and prejudices against those who suffer. We need to understand that *anyone* can become overwhelmed, anxious, depressed, or even dissociate from reality just to survive. Some may even have a genetic predisposition to depression or anxiety, with or without stress. Some may be prone to depression under stress, as with a sensitive nervous system. And many, unable to cope, may use psychotic defense mechanisms to survive.

Recovery from depression, like recovery from pain, involves finding a balance between under doing and overdoing, and reclaiming all aspects of life, including one's spiritual side (not to be confused with going to church). Practices such as prayer, meditation, daily exercise, and biofeedback may restore such balance, release the damaging effects of stress, and allow for the needed mindful changes. I discuss these activities in detail in my next book, *Heal Thyself! What You Can Do to Recover from Chronic Pain and Depression.*

For those who are religious, a strong religious faith may be helpful—if it is not destroyed by the depression and if it does not contribute to negative voices of depression like guilt, fear, and self-loathing. For those who are not religious, there are many different ways to manage stress and loss, to be more creative, and to reach out to others to be more fully human. Meditation may be helpful here. And when traumatic events overwhelm us and interfere with our ability to cope or to use meditation or prayer, medical treatments and the doctor-patient relationship become crucial in encouraging a return to healthy living.

Addressing Negative Thinking

In the final analysis, depression, anxiety, fear, anger, guilt, and loneliness have a lot to do with how much pain is felt in any given situation. Furthermore, chronic pain gives rise to emotional states and behaviors such as despair, hopelessness, helplessness, inactivity, social withdrawal, and loss of interest in activities that can distract from pain. These complicate, and may worsen, the original problem. Chronic pain leads to changes in behavior, such as walking with a limp, using a cane, or taking pills. While some of these changes may be useful, some may become the focus of life to the exclusion of more important things.

Along with depression, chronic pain may give rise to negative thinking that reinforces the status quo: "I'm sick," "I'm disabled," "I'm too old," "I don't have enough faith," "I can't get better," "If I move, I'll hurt myself," and so on. Recognizing and changing the negative messages is one important goal of treatment in chronic pain conditions and in depression itself.

Many people become depressed after loss, trauma, or illness. This is true for victims of war and for the many who live traumatic, difficult, and threatened lives. We see the incidence of depression increase after catastrophes, in people who are poor and constantly under stress, in communities threatened with constant violence, and in soldiers after terrible battles. Some of these depressions are called post-traumatic stress disorder (PTSD). Many soldiers returning from Iraq (and now Afghanistan) have suffered chronic pain problems, *even though they have suffered no physical injuries.*[30] These soldiers have become inactive, discouraged about their futures, and depressed. No one is immune.

CHAPTER FIFTEEN

STARTING A PROGRAM FOR
CHRONIC PAIN AND DEPRESSION

If I had not been already been meditating, I would cer-
tainly have had to start. I've treated my own depression
for many years with exercise and meditation, and I've
found that to be a tremendous help.
—Judy Collins

In 1993, I began working with the physical therapy department and with several other physicians at Cooper Green to create a program to address the needs of patients with a mix of depression and chronic pain. Many of these patients also had serious medical problems, so part of our challenge was to coordinate care with the physicians or treatment staff working with these other illnesses. We were concerned that many patients were falling through the cracks and not receiving optimum treatment for anything. Depressed patients frequently do not follow through, and those in pain may be more concerned with getting pills to relieve the pain than with treating their serious illness.

Although at the time we failed to achieve a combined clinic because many of the physicians left or moved on to other things, I did add a second group therapy and a program devoted to those with depression and pain.

A friend, Jane Trechsel, volunteered to do yoga with the group and later wrote a book (*A Morning Cup of Yoga*[31]) that presents a daily yoga routine anyone can do and benefit from. She also recorded a relaxation CD she called *Just Rest*, which she shared with the group. She initiated simple breathing exercises and different meditations. Because I could see how powerful these practices were in helping patients improve, I took over the meditation and guided imagery with the group when she left.

A number of other volunteers came from the community to offer patients alternative and complementary therapies such as meditation, yoga, massage, and exercise (chair aerobics and swimming). The YMCA and Saint Vincent's Hospital allowed our patients to participate in water aerobics at their facilities without cost. Some chiropractors were willing to volunteer their services, but the medical staff at Cooper Green was uncomfortable with that. An acupuncturist was also willing to work with some of our patients, but the state would only allow physicians to practice acupuncture in a hospital setting.

I had always encouraged patients to develop their own exercise and stretching routines at home. Now a physical therapist would meet with them to evaluate what they were doing and add to their daily plans. Having patients begin *something* was the key, as was getting the physical therapists to set small, realistic goals with patients that involved the whole body rather than go for big changes in targeted areas in the short period allowed for therapy. Many patients came back amazed at how fast small amounts of exercise and stretching helped their pain and their moods.

The real challenge was getting people to start doing daily exercise, no matter how little. I used my own story with exercise, and the stories of other patients who had seen the benefit of exercise, to encourage them. I also loved to tell the story of the sixty-nine-year-old man who was admitted to the hospital with obesity, hypertension, diabetes, depression, and arthritis. He was put on an exercise routine, and at eighty-nine he

---

[31] Jane Goad Trechsel, *A Morning Cup of Yoga* (China: Crane Hill Publishers, Inc., 2002).

was still running in marathons: *no obesity, no hypertension, no diabetes, no depression, and no arthritis!* Ah! The miracle of exercise!

In the group, I tied the guided imagery I used during the meditations to the issues discussed in the group that day. That allowed me to do some teaching and modeling as well. After allowing patients to release tension by talking about their frustrations, I would use the meditation to release the tension held in the muscles. The guided meditation also gave me a chance to slip in some new ideas or reinforce old ones. Without fail, patients reported at the end that their pain was better. This encouraged other patients to try meditation at home. I persuaded patients to experiment with different images during the meditation to see what helped most to manage stress and high-pain times. Some found that imagining themselves by a stream, listening to the water flow by, was the most helpful. Others preferred the bright light that came down over their heads and focused on areas where they held pain or tension. Some patients had difficulty imagining anything for themselves, while others came up with ideas that worked even better than what I had thought of.

Johnson Porter had severe diabetes with painful neuropathy. He consumed a lot of medicines, including opiates for pain. He had been forced to retire because he was too sick to work. Johnson was amazed at how much the group and other activities had helped him. "You know, these breathing exercises allow me to walk further in the morning and take less medicine than I did before. I use it not only during the day when I have more pain, but anytime I want to be more active." His *walking meditation* allowed him to do more.

After a year, Johnson began talking about his life in group. "You know, this meditation is powerful stuff. I'm not the same man I was a year ago. In fact, I don't think I'd have lost all those good wives I had if I'd been doing this meditating all my life!" Johnson had discovered on his own, the power of meditation to make us more mindful of how we relate to others and how we deal with anger.

Susie Rogers also found meditation a powerful help. "I find that using different themes with the meditation helps me deal with the pain and other problems in my life," she said. Apparently, patients were using meditation as a kind of self-hypnosis or dissociation to help manage their pain; Susie had a special routine she used to get relief when the pain became unbearable. Susie had found a way to use her considerable imagination help her manage her life.

As other patients continued with the relaxation and breathing exercises, they began noticing more about themselves. Laretha Jones was a thirty-nine-year-old woman who had never married and had never been employed for long. She was still traumatized by being brought up by an aunt who did not want her. As a result, Laretha had been in jail and psychiatric hospitals repeatedly for being out of control. She left school in the sixth grade. To most people, Laretha looked like a street person— clothes disheveled, hair unbrushed, most of her teeth missing. She was sent to see me for treatment of pain and depression. Laretha had pain in her right shoulder and had to move her arm around constantly to keep it from hurting.

Looking at her right arm and hand, she said, "I don't know why I have to keep moving. I have to keep moving that arm, or it hurts. The doctor says I have some arthritis in that shoulder, but it sure hurts." Laretha rubbed it and asked me how I would help her.

"I would really like to have you come to the group I have for people with chronic pain. I think it can help you."

Laretha thought for a minute. "I don't know," she said. "I can't always get away. I live with my brother; at least, he's supposed to look after me, but I can't always depend on him." She agreed to take medicine for depression and come when she could.

Laretha was a good group member. She spoke right up when something did not make sense to her, and she worked hard to do the exercises. One day I saw her struggle to relax during the relaxation exercise and grow more agitated instead. "I couldn't relax," she said afterward. "I couldn't stop moving my arm."

"Just remember what you have been talking about in group," I said. "How angry you are at the man who raped you and also at your brother for not protecting you. The exercise helps you get in touch with what is really going on with you. You're too angry to be calm at the moment."

She looked at me in astonishment. "Do you mean that I keep popping my arm so I won't go pop that man and end up in jail again?" Her insight was marvelous.

It was six months before I saw her again. She had been having a difficult time, evicted from home and living on the street, but she was beaming from ear to ear when she came in. "I'm never going to jail again," she told the group. "Whenever I start to get mad, I just do my breathing exercises and let the feeling go." She still had some pain in her arm, but she had stopped moving it and was doing better. "I'm even doing the walking you told me to do," she said proudly. Anger has its place to defend us from assault, but revenge tends to get us into trouble.

Most patient stories were not so dramatic, but nonetheless, it was wonderful to see people saddled with a difficult existence find ways to get back some control over their emotions and their lives. Hector Abbot had been forced to retire from his management job at a Piggly Wiggly market because of severe heart disease. He had come to Cooper Green because he had been impressed with the care his father had received there. He had been more successful in life than most of the other patients, so I was afraid he would not come to group, but he did, and he was surprised at how much the group and its activities helped him. "I couldn't believe that using breathing and relaxation could make such a difference to my pain! I must tense up a lot when I start to hurt. I know I find myself tensing up when I just think about the pain." After he got better, he volunteered to help others who were going through the disability process. He also assisted us with the smoking cessation part of the program.

Herman Tuttle had been a successful accountant until someone nearly killed him on the highway. Herman had had many surgeries and knew more were planned for the future before he'd be able to walk again. His medical insurance had been great at the time of the accident, but now over eight years later he was out of insurance and just barely through the disability process. "They turned me down the first three times I applied." he sighed as he talked. "They just didn't seem to understand how barely walking, in constant pain, I could not go back to being an accountant. My father has spent all of his savings paying my medical bills because my insurance would only cover two years if I wasn't working. It's a crazy system. It won't cover you when you really need it. Thank heavens for Cooper Green." Herman was astounded at how much the meditation helped his pain. "I guess I'm still angry with that trucking company trying to weasel out of responsibility for what they did to me. Just because their driver died doesn't mean it was my fault. No one wants to take responsibility for anything these days. The police report was clear." Herman became one of our best helpers. He didn't always feel up to coming, but when he did he was always ready to assist others. "I can help those going through the disability process. I certainly know the ins and outs all too well."

Jon Kabat-Zinn, author of *Full Catastrophe Living*, wrote about the power of mindfulness meditation to change all aspects of one's life.[32] Even in the rather primitive setting at Cooper Green, patients were able to take these simple exercises and turn their lives around.

Dealing with Resistance

Some patients coming to group had trouble making changes to help themselves. Even some of the most successful patients, those who had prospered in business before being derailed by illness or injury, had difficulty accepting the need for stretching and exercise. Tom Allen came regularly to group, but he always had an objection. "I can't believe the doctors can't fix this pain. There must be something they can do to make it go away!" He went on, "You said I would hurt less if I distracted myself with something interesting or absorbing, but every time I work in my shop for any length of time, my back hurts me more!"

Even though I doubted Tom would be able to hear me, I welcomed a chance to explain further. I knew there would be someone else in the group with the same question who might. "Interesting activity distracts you from the pain as long as the activity is not putting an added strain on your injured part. If it does, the increased pain may be a message

---

[32] Jon Kabat-Zinn, *Full Catastrophe Living: Using the Wisdom of Your Body and Mind to Face Stress, Pain, and Illness* (New York: Delacorte, 1990).

that it's time to take a break, move and stretch a little, or do something else for a while and come back to the activity that hurts you later. If you have been standing, maybe you need to sit for a while, and vice versa. The key here is to experiment and find what works best for you with your particular limitations." Tom still looked skeptical, but I could see a window open for some of the others.

Roland Maise spoke up. "I've been planting a garden," he said, shifting in his chair and looking excited. "I can't do a lot at one time, but I plan in my head how to get it all done, then I plan each section before I do any actual work. Planning the garden distracts me too. It's much better than sitting around watching TV, feeling sorry for myself! My wife's been bugging me for years to plant something and it looks like we'll have tomatoes and corn at least this year."

Imagination! How often I saw how imagination could fuel progress and failure to imagine a goal, be it more activity, a completed project or one in stages, could hold people back. Material success in life did not seem to correlate with having the best imagination. Sometimes imagination was a gift to those who had struggled and overcome the most.

CHAPTER SIXTEEN

THE UNFOLDING ADDICTION PROBLEM

To array a man's will against his sickness is the supreme art of medicine.
—Henry Ward Beecher

Working with chronic pain patients at Cooper Green, I found that I was seeing more and more addicts who were not recognized as such by their doctors. Take the case of Joe Banks. Joe had sustained an injury to his left hip, and his X-ray looked terrible. His internist was convinced that Joe had a lot of pain and gave him stronger and stronger opiates. The internist eventually sent Joe to me for the treatment of depression. Joe had symptoms of depression, but mainly, he was addicted to opiates. Joe "lost" prescriptions over and over. He frequently went to the emergency room or to his doctor for shots because the pain was so bad; he always wanted stronger and stronger medicines. Even when he did not have the money to take care of his family, he used what he had to buy medication not covered by insurance or Cooper Green. He was looking for a bigger bang, no matter who it hurt.

When I first saw Joe in a group of people with chronic pain problems, he stood out by a mile. He would sit in a corner writhing in pain; no one else in the group even looked uncomfortable. When I asked the group members to relax, Joe would increase the amount of tension in his muscles and eventually say he had to go find his doctor and get a shot. It was obvious to me and to the other members of the group what Joe was doing, but his doctor was so convinced of Joe's pain that no input from me, and not even Joe's wife's statement that he was abusing his medicine, would prevent his young doctor from prescribing more and more opiates.

"Sam, can't you see how Joe is manipulating you?" I said to the doctor one day. "His wife has even admitted to me he's abusing drugs. He is going to different emergency rooms to get medicine."

Sam shook his head while I spoke. "Joe had a broken back; you should see his X-ray. I've watched him when he didn't know I was there, and he's still writhing in pain. I may have to put him in the hospital again to break the pain cycle," he said.

It did no good to say, "But people with chronic pain don't writhe. They may not even look as if they have any pain at all! That writhing is Joe putting on!"

Eventually, Joe died of an overdose, and his wife admitted to this doctor that they had both been getting drugs from a number of sources. She asked him for help getting off the drugs herself. Joe's wife also came to see me after he died. "I can't believe the doctors didn't see through Joe's manipulations. He'd take that X-ray of his to any emergency room in town, and they always gave him just about anything he wanted. He didn't like coming to you, because you saw through his lies. We were both very stupid. He might have gotten away with it if he hadn't tried to get high by grinding up the stuff and putting it in a syringe." The wife had agreed to get into drug treatment because of her children. "I was never as bad as him, anyway," she said.

At that time, I did not realize that it would be the problem with addicts in the hospital that would give me the opportunity to implement a full program for patients with depression, pain, illness, and addiction.

Opiate Prescribing Practices Contribute to the Addiction Problem

In assessing the extent of the addiction problem at the hospital, I interviewed most of the physicians about their philosophy of opiate use as well as nurses and other staff about opiate use in the hospital. What

I discovered was striking: the quantity and type of opiates patients received had more to do with the attitude of the physician than what was wrong with the patient!

Some physicians refused to provide opiates at all for fear of creating addicts or of being manipulated by current addicts. Others managed medications well enough, but often, that was all they offered to treat the patient's pain. At one time, they might have sent a patient for brief courses of physical therapy, but they did not tie medication use to exercise or encourage patients to be more active. Thus, the message was, "The pill will do away with the pain," not "Recovery from this pain involves moving and stretching; use the medicine to help you be more active and you will get better."

Still other physicians regularly gave out whatever pain medicines patients wanted, inadvertently enabling many patients to abuse opiates. For the most part, these enablers were supplying a population of drug addicts without being aware of it. Some of the most caring physicians were blind to how they were being manipulated. The community knew exactly which physicians supplied opiates, so addicts lined up to see them. The nurses knew all about which doctors gave out too many pills and which patients came looking for a fix, but this information did not always get back to the physicians. At one point, locks had to be put on the medical clinic door just so patients would not walk in to ask Dr. X for another prescription.

Selling opiate prescriptions was big business for many patients. Many would come to the hospital, get opiates, and have them sold before getting back on the bus. Many of the staff I interviewed thought that selling pills was the only means for some patients to get food and shelter. Many of the nurses and doctors I interviewed thought there was no way to address the problem of selling prescriptions, because it was so ingrained in the culture of Cooper Green.

It reminded me of an educational game I had played at Leadership Birmingham, an organization aimed at education and building community. We were dealt picture cards at random; the cards could be traded for "money." Some trades made you richer, and some got you nowhere. Those in the top third with the most money made the rules about the next round. Those with the most assets made rules that benefitted themselves and made it even harder for those at the bottom to move up.

I could see what was happening after the first round, so on the next trade, I gave all my assets to someone else on the bottom: something to trade up with. Then, since no one checked to see how many points we had, I lied about my points when I wrote them on my card. That moved me up with my friend.

During the debriefing session, we talked about our experiences with the game. Everyone seemed surprised that I would lie. "You, of all people," someone said. Even the leaders were surprised, saying they had never had anyone lie before.

I laughed. "I could see that the game was set up to demonstrate how people at the top contrive to favor themselves and make it harder for others to move up. That challenged me to find a way to move up anyway." People without power do not play by the rules, because the rules do not work for them!

The Challenge of Opiates and Addiction

The more pain patients I saw, the more addicts I saw who had serious medical problems. Addicts are at high risk for a number of serious diseases, like the AIDS virus and hepatitis C, because of unprotected sex and dirty needles. Also, they are prone to injuries from fights, accidents, or falls. Because of sporadic work histories, they often lack medical insurance. These patients needed help with their pain and addiction while they were undergoing medical treatment for other conditions. Having them continue to take drugs from the street increased the likelihood of dangerous drug interactions.

Roy James, who was sent to me by his physician early in my time at Cooper Green, exemplified the problem. Roy was a wiry man in his mid-forties who had depression. He had worked on and off in the past, but since he had hepatitis C and a bad leg, he could not work anymore. I pressed him about his work, but he was vague. From the outset it was clear to me that Roy was an addict who just wanted pills. His chart said he was suffering from depression. There was no mention of addiction.

"Why are you asking me all these questions?" Roy asked, obviously irritated. "I just need something for pain and for my nerves."

"Tell me about the problem with your nerves," I followed, not responding to his irritation.

"What do you mean, 'Tell me about your nerves?' If you don't know what nerves are like, how can you help me?" He turned halfway around in his chair as if to change the subject.

"How long have you had problems with your nerves?" I continued mildly.

"What difference does that make?" he threw back. "I've always had trouble with my nerves, but now it's worse than ever, and the doctor won't give me anything more for pain or my nerves until you see me."

"What do you take for pain and your nerves?" I pursued.

"Any damn thing I can get!" he said. "How do you expect me to live like this without some help? If I can't get it here, I know where I can get it."

"What helps you the most?" I continued.

"Valiums or Lortabs are best," he reported. "But I can't always get them."

"When did you last have some, and what did you have?" I responded.

"What do you mean, what did I have? What difference does that make? I need something now."

This conversation continued, revealing a pattern of street drug use dating back many years, along with alcohol abuse and admission to various drug treatment programs and twelve-step programs. Roy grew angrier and more and more belligerent as we talked. He denied having any problem other than suffering from pain and nerves.

"You need something for your nerves that won't conflict with your treatment for hepatitis C," I said, trying to arrive at a reasonable way to help this man. "Let me discuss this with your doctors and then see what is the best approach. You must not drink, or take Lortabs because it contains Tylenol and they will damage your liver, so we should find some pain medicine that will help you but won't hurt you or interfere with your treatment here."

"You mean you're not going to give me something now?" He stood up. "I should have gone back to the emergency room. I can always depend on them for a few pills." He stormed out.

Roy was not in withdrawal from drugs or alcohol, which would have necessitated an intervention, and since he just wanted pills, he probably would go to the street. A coordinated program with his treating physicians so that he could get opiates or tranquilizers from us rather than from the street would have benefited him, but I had no such program in place then. I felt helpless to do anything but suggest to his physician giving him safe tranquilizers and pain medication to keep him off the street while he was going through treatment. Later, I was able to develop a program for addicts who had pain and other medical conditions that could assist Roy during the acute phase of his treatment for hepatitis C. It would have given Roy a better chance to get into a treatment program to address his addiction as well.

Finally, the drug problem in the clinic got so out of control that the hospital administration stepped in to centralize the evaluation, treatment, and monitoring of patients who had complex problems involving pain, drug addiction, anxiety, and depression. In 2003, after ten years of working with chronic pain patients, I was asked to put together a multidisciplinary pain program for the hospital and to assist with the problem of addicts. I assume that the practice of patients selling prescriptions to pay for food, lodging, and other needs is such a vast social phenomenon that it continues to this day.

CHAPTER SEVENTEEN

PREPARING FOR THE NEW ENDORPHIN CLINIC: A DEEPER LOOK AT ADDICTION

Among the remedies which it has pleased the Almighty
God to give to man to relieve his sufferings, none is so
universal and so efficacious as opium.
—Thomas Sydenham, MD

In preparing for the new clinic, I talked with all the medical providers who treated pain at Cooper Green, including the orthopedist, the rheumatologist, the neurologist, and the anesthesiologist who ran the clinic for pain blocks. I also spoke with many of the nurses and others about how the existing system worked and what could make it better. I searched the literature for information about pain programs. I talked with a number of pain clinics in town, physicians treating pain and addiction, and the head of the UAB drug rehabilitation program. Most people were generous with their time and suggestions. Only a few were reluctant to share their secrets for fear we would be competition! Dr. Dan Doleys allowed me to ask questions and spend time in his pain clinic. In the end, I put together a program for Cooper Green based on all of the information I had gleaned from these sources, modified by my experience seeing patients in the Cooper Green setting.

A Clinic by Any Other Name

Planning for the pain clinic, I looked for a name that would represent an approach to chronic pain that was different from the traditional medical one of pills and shots. I decided to call it the Endorphin Clinic. I was attracted to the word *endorphin* rather than *pain,* because it conveyed the right story for our patients. I wanted to encourage all the positive activities that increased endorphins and brought about healing from within, while reinforcing what each individual must do to recover his or her own life and health. It was the body's own capacity to heal that I wanted to tap in this clinic. Also, using *endorphin* instead of *pain* in the clinic's name meant that patients did not have to keep hurting to continue getting treatment there.

Educating Physicians about the Use of Opiates and Addiction

As part of assessing what the Endorphin Clinic could reasonably offer to address the addiction problem in the hospital, I asked the hospital pharmacy to list all opiate prescriptions for a month. When the hospital administration and medical staff saw the results, they were shocked at the number of prescriptions being written. While the administration spoke with some physicians directly about the number of opiate prescriptions they were writing, presumably supplying addicts, I decided to focus on a better approach to pain management than just medication, by offering educational programs to all the medical providers about addiction, opiate use, and all aspects of the treatment of chronic pain. This gave me an added chance to educate medical providers about patients with sensitive nervous systems and cut down on the indiscriminate use of opiates by telling them how the Endorphin Clinic would assist them with the management of patients with chronic pain, depression and addiction.

So....What does it mean to be an Addict? What is Addiction?

Working with physicians and patients in pain, I realized how poorly the whole issue of opiates and addiction was understood, so I invited a number of addiction and pain specialists in the community to speak to the medical staff. I thought it was important to understand that the tendency to addiction has as much to do with the person as it does the substance. True, some drugs are more addictive than others, and certainly opiates

encourage compulsive use, but the user's individual traits and characteristics make him or her more or less prone to addiction. Addiction and
alcoholism run in families. Adoption studies have shown that children
are more apt to behave like their biological parents than their adoptive
ones when it comes to drugs and alcohol.[33]

How Opiates Promote Overuse

Anyone who takes an opiate daily for two weeks or longer becomes
physically dependent and will have some withdrawal symptoms if
the drug is stopped abruptly. Also after two weeks the opiate is not
as effective as it was in the beginning. This is the result of tolerance having developed. This can happen with many other medicines
and is the reason why one should taper off (decrease gradually) most
medicine if it has been taken for a while. (It's also why the side effect
of medicines go away over time.) Most of the time as we heal after
surgery or an injury we take less and less medicine tapering ourselves
off naturally.

When tolerance develops to the pain relieving aspects of the opiates,
patients have to take more medicine to get the same pain relief. It also
means they will hurt more when the effect of the opiate wears off. So the
tendency may be to take more and more medicine to get a greater effect.
Medicines have a number of effects, and we do not develop tolerance to
all of the effects of the drug. We do not develop tolerance to the lethal
effects of the opiates.

Abuse is Different From Addiction

Abuse means using enough of a substance to create a social or physical
problem. Generally speaking, the likelihood of abuse increases when
people are under stress, as well as when they are around others drinking
or using drugs. Most American soldiers in Vietnam, perhaps as many

---

[33] Louis Goodman and Alfred Gilman, *The Pharmacological Basis of Therapeutics*
(New York: McGraw-Hill, 1970).

as 80 percent, abused heroin and other drugs, but when they returned home, only one in eight continued to seek out drugs.[34]

Being addicted is more than abuse. Addiction involves the pursuit of the drug even when it is causing physical, emotional, social, occupational, or legal difficulties. At least half of Americans abuse drugs or alcohol sometime in their lives, but about 8 to 10 percent of the population is addicted and cannot stop taking a drug, even if it is causing major problems.

Problems in Physicians' Approach to Addicts

Cultures choose which addictions are socially acceptable and which need censure. In America, addictions to caffeine and, until recently, nicotine, were acceptable because these addictions increase productivity. Marijuana on the other hand has many beneficial effects, but it makes those who use it regularly too laid back for our culture. The young who use it regularly cease to be energetic and ambitious, perhaps from the brain damage that can be caused by regular use. Alcohol causes both physical and mental damage and more social problems than heroin, but has proved impossible to outlaw. Heroin and cocaine on the other hand, were drugs originally found in minority communities so they have attracted the most censure. Physicians have absorbed the cultural attitudes about drugs with the rest of the country.

Cultural attitudes about drugs are only one reason physicians have had a hard time dealing with addiction. The fact that addicts lie and manipulate the system to get drugs is a stumbling block for many physicians, especially if they have trouble detecting lying in others. Some physicians even judge lying itself as immoral though it is part of the syndrome of addiction, and something everyone does. Then the association of criminal behavior with addiction and the criminalization of certain addictions have been a major stumbling block for many physicians. In addition, most physicians don't have access to the type of programs needed to manage their patient's addictions within a medical setting.

---

[34] S. Peele, "What is Addiction and How Do People Get It: Diseasing America." (1995) [Electronic Version] The Stanton Peele Addiction Website, 6, p22

Moreover, many doctors have blind spots that make them useless in treating an addict population. All physicians working with addicts need to be aware of their blind spots, and know whether they tend to prescribe too much or too little opiate pain medicine. If they do deal with addicts, they should work with a team of professionals so they can minimize the effect of their biases and maximize the chance that someone can reach the addict and improve his or her chances of getting reasonable treatment.

Some doctors feel uncomfortable with the current demand that they manage chronic pain problems; once, pain management was confined to certain specialties. Since the focus on pain as the fifth vital sign, along with pulse, respiration, temperature and blood pressure doctors are forced to focus more on pain which tends to lead to more prescriptions for pain medication. Changing attitudes about the use of pain medication in those with chronic pain not of cancer origin, has not helped either.

Problems with the Current Approach to Opiate Use

The attitudes toward opiate use are always changing. I have noted that in my youth, doctors were very stingy with opiates because they were afraid of causing addiction. Now we have gone to the other extreme; too many opiates are prescribed.

The Risks and Benefits of Taking Opiates

Treatment of pain brought on by life-threatening illnesses is important to survival. During a heart attack, or after major burns or severe injury, pain places too much stress on the heart. Physicians treat this kind of pain with opiates to prevent the deadly triangle of anxiety, depression, and sleeplessness. These are the symptoms that constitute suffering and lead to increased sickness (morbidity) and death (mortality). Today we recognize that both pain and depression increase the risk for having a heart attack. Opiates are valuable drugs to combat these stresses.

Treatment of Chronic Pain with Opiates: The Goal Is to Improve Function

In 1997, when I interviewed the medical staff at Cooper Green about the way they prescribed opiates, most of the physicians believed that doctors give opiates to make patients *feel* better. They did not realize that doctors really give opiates so patients will *do* better: start getting up, moving around, getting back to their normal life. The only way to avoid being misled by patients (or by their own biases and preconceived ideas, for that matter), is to focus on function—what the patients *do*—not on how patients feel. Sometimes function and how patients feel go together: as patients feel better, they get up and go back to their normal, active routine. But that is not always the case.

Even with the same injuries, illnesses, or stresses, some patients report a lot of pain, while others complain very little. By looking at how opiates help patients work, exercise, maintain healthy sexual relationships, and get out with their families and friends, physicians will find it easier not to over- or underuse opiates or other strong pain medications. Too many physicians prescribe pills without assessing whether the pain is worse because the person does not stretch regularly or exercise enough to keep muscles flexible! Tying the use of opiates to exercise and increased activity means patients are doing what they need to do to get better permanently. Having patients take daily opiates without being more active or involved in normal work and relationships activities, the doctor may set up a potentially dangerous situation with the opiates, and also cheat the patient of an opportunity to learn the importance of stretching and exercise for managing ongoing painful conditions.

Information from Families Keeps the Focus on Function

Talking to a patient's family provides information about how the patient is functioning and any compulsive use of their medication including medications for sleep, anxiety, and depression. Many times, family members have told me that a patient is overmedicated, even while the patient was telling me he or she felt fine. The goal should be for a patient to *function better*, rather than just to feel fine. This is true even with antidepressants that are non-addicting. One reason for this is that patients tend do better *before* they feel better. It's by doing better that they end up feeling better—not by just lying around taking pills.

One of the speaker I asked to talk about opiates was Dr. Jack Waites, an addictionologist from the rehabilitation program at Bradford Health Services in Birmingham. He spoke to us about opiate use. Imagine my surprise when he pointed out that *opiates increase the amount of pain experienced over time*—and also reduce the taker's awareness of new physical problems, like burns or infected teeth! He added, "*Six weeks after opiates have been withdrawn, as many as 80 percent become pain free even in the addict population.* That's especially true if the person has sustained an injury that has since healed."

I had known that all patients being evaluated for pain pump implants in the brain had to be withdrawn from opiates for six weeks to assess their true pain level since opiates can induce hyperalgesia (increased pain), but I had not realized how many patients actually have more pain *because of* daily opiate use. For some, this *opiate-induced hyperalgesia* begins in the early weeks of taking opiates and may be confused with tolerance.[35] Impressed as I was by these experts' information, convincing doctors to give patients more rehabilitation and fewer opiates proved harder than I could have imagined.

The Downsides of Regular Opiate Use

The negative effects of chronic opiate use include chronic constipation, sedation, and sleepiness. There may be increased danger of infection, because along with shrinkage of the thymus and spleen, B and T cell function in the immune system are suppressed, and the effectiveness of phagocytes in eliminating harmful bacteria and fungi is decreased. Chronic opiate use impairs endocrine function as well, and may lead to hypogonadism (decreased function of the testes or ovaries).

---

[35] See Chapter Twenty.

In addition to the risk of addiction with continued use, as tolerance develops, pain increases (a phenomenon now known as opiate-induced hyperalgesia). This results in failure to attend to new pain signals that might be important.

Opiate-Induced Hyperalgesia

As I have noted, over time regular opiate use gradually increases the amount of pain the user experiences. There are several reasons for this; some are understood and others are still being worked out. The body metabolizes some opiates—specifically, morphine, oxycodone, fentanyl, and hydromorphone (Dilaudid)—into substances that make pain worse. These metabolized by-products become an important consideration when they accumulate and are not eliminated from the body. Different opiates attach to the nervous system using combinations of the three opiate receptors: delta, mu, and theta. Switching from one opiate to another may avoid some of the chronic use problems with any one opiate, but this isn't straight forward. And one is always wisest to use a multi dimentional approach to managing pain.

Any Medicine Used for Pain May Cause Rebound Pain

Another reason for the increased pain with chronic opiate use is its *rebound* phenomenon. As pain medication wears off, it causes a withdrawal that actually leads to more pain. This also happens with some of the drugs used to treat migraine headaches. Caffeine is often an ingredient in migraine medications; it alone can give rise to rebound, or caffeine-withdrawal, headaches. If pain is recurrent and persistent, it's wise to *taper off all medications* and any other substances that have been taken for any length of time.

However, getting patients off opiates means educating them not to go back to the big doses of opiate or other medication they were taking before they stopped. Large doses of opiate can be lethal if one has not built up a tolerance to the drug. Many young addicts die this way, taking their former dose to get high after a period of abstinence.

Stress Messages that Increase Pain: Opiates as Blockers

Unlike other painkillers, opiates alleviate pain that is accompanied by fear, stress, and portentous dread of injury or disease. It appears that opiates work on the brain's interpretation of pain. They block signals to the pain receptors that say, "You're in real trouble," which explains why they have no effect in a laboratory setting where there is no fear of permanent damage.

Opiate Instructions

Doctors need to tell patients: "Use the opiate to break bad pain cycles and to help you continue to exercise and stretch daily, work, or have sex when otherwise the pain might interfere." This is far more effective than for a physician to say to take it merely "as needed." Doctors should also encourage having a plan for days when the pain is worse, either because the weather is bad, or the patient has been overdoing or not stretching an exercising enough. When less activity has caused muscles to tighten up, it's better to loosen up the muscles by mild exercise and stretching. A sample plan for bad pain days is described in Appendix E.

Looking for Depression

To insure that an opiate isn't being used to treat depression instead of pain, any person with chronic pain who is on opiates should also be watched for depression and—if necessary—treated with medication for depression and talk therapy, preferably in a group setting.

CHAPTER EIGHTEEN

HARM REDUCTION: A PROGRAM FOR ADDICTS

Nowhere in the world, despite the application of every
conceivable form of prevention and treatment measure
including the most draconian means of intimidation
(long term incarceration, hanging, beheading, torture)
has been preventive in stopping illicit drug use.
—RG Newman, MD

Over the years at Cooper Green, many patients with drug or alcohol problems were sent to me for the treatment of depression. Many of them were on opiates for pain, but all too often, no mention of their addiction history was made in the medical record.

The treatment program we developed for addicts at Cooper Green, in conjunction with Dr. Norm Huggins and the University of Alabama drug program, was designed to maximize the chances of addicts going through medical treatment successfully and without the added risks of street drugs. Our goal was harm reduction—that is, to reduce sickness and death from illness and addiction.

The concept of harm reduction is borrowed from the experience of methadone programs, where it was discovered that patients are more apt to die if they are discharged from the program for relapsing (using drugs). It is better to recognize that part of addiction is using drugs, re-lapsing, and then lying about it, and it is far more productive to get these patients back into treatment, intensify their drug rehabilitation, and help them get back on track than to treat them like criminals because they use drugs and lie.

This, however, is not the same as letting patients manipulate the doctor to get more pain medicine. The goal for the person out of control from the use of a drug, any drug, is abstinence from the addicting drug. The *key to success resides in how the patient gets to abstinence.*

It is important to realize that initially, addicts may need *more* opiate medication than other chronic pain patients, because not only are they able to tolerate larger doses, it makes them focus less on their need for drugs so they can focus on the rest of their lives, and participate in rehabilitation aspects of the program. Denying opiates to addicts initially sets up an immediate conflict that may be counterproductive: as with Roy James, they leave to get more drugs, and when they cannot get medical drugs, they go to the street. Giving them opiates, such as a long-acting one like methadone, relieves the pressure of that need. The patient has time to develop trust in the doctor and become willing to give up seeking drugs from the street, a practice that is especially dangerous if the patient is undergoing medical treatment. At Cooper Green, some physicians were already prescribing opiates for their addict patients to get them away from street drugs while they were being treated for cancer, AIDS, or hepatitis C.

The Opiate's Potential for Causing Addiction

Of patients who are given opiates for pain, most easily give up the drug when the pain is gone. Fewer than 1 percent will become addicted when an opiate is given short term. Even among patients who are known to be addicts before they are treated with opiates for acute injury or post-surgical pain, only 10 percent will become addicted. Even with the chronic use of opiates to treat pain, only about 50 percent of those with a history of polysubstance abuse(multiple drug) become addicted to the opiate. So initially, it does not matter which opiates a patient takes. Doctors can safely give a patient what the patient wants. A few doses won't an addict make!

Opiate Treatment in Addicts

Addicts whose drug of choice is something other than an opiate are more likely to be able to manage opiates given for pain, even if their addiction to another substance is out of control. This means that doctors should not be reluctant to treat those who can benefit from opiates simply because they fear that prescribing an opiate will bring on a patient's addiction.

On the other hand, just prescribing opiates to addicts to keep them from getting street drugs while they are treated for cancer or hepatitis C, without getting them involved in a rehabilitation program at the same time, means they can be lost to addiction after treatment of the illness is complete. Realistically, sometimes just giving medications is the best we doctors can do, but using the opportunity to build on the doctor-patient relationship and getting patients involved in the recovery program may give the addicted patient a chance to get his or her life back.

Many addicts were neglected as children and never had good role models for handling life's difficulties. Some have never been cared about as much as they are with the intense treatment within a medical setting. So, the doctor-patient relationship may not only keep patients involved in doing difficult personal work, but it can also see them through detox from opiates and other drugs. A strong doctor-patient relationship can be a powerful tool to encourage addicts to get passionate about doing something with their lives other than drugs. It may give them their only chance to escape the drug world.

Treating Addicts with Opiates

Even addicts with chronic pain and no serious medical illnesses do better if they are not withdrawn from opiates too quickly, because they tend to resist substance abuse treatment, saying they have a pain, not a drug problem, and may just leave. The doctor's first task, then, is to get the patient involved in the pain recovery program that includes daily exercise and stretching, meditation, group therapy to deal with life issues, family therapy, and perhaps job skills training. To convince patients to follow through, doctors need trusting and understanding relationships with them. This, plus some pain management skills are especially important when the time comes to withdraw opiates to assess the true pain level. Convincing patients that the opiates are causing, worsening, or contributing to their pain rather than lessening it become easier if a full rehabilitation program is in place and patients can trust doctors not to abandon them to their pain.

Once patients develop some pain-control skills and trust in the doctor, the physician can withdraw the opiates without causing the patient the sense of loss he or she might have experienced if the opiates had been stopped early in the treatment, before the pain recovery program. Patients with addiction issues will become obvious going through the pain recovery program, and their addictions can be addressed directly. But, unless a well-structured program exists to assist outpatients with withdrawal symptoms (using clonidine, for example), inpatient detoxification is necessary.

The greatest challenge in our clinic was educating doctors and staff about opiate use, addiction, and the importance of group therapy for learning new pain management skills and confronting self-defeating behavior. Addicts and others exhibiting self-defeating behavior tend to do best in groups where they can be confronted by peers who recognize when they are lying to themselves and who can encourage them to make the necessary changes.

Since many addicts just wanted to get opiates rather than take part in drug treatment or pain rehab, we needed a program where the staff worked together consistently to encourage rehabilitation. Otherwise, patients would manipulate the system just to get the drugs. However, implementing a consistent front proved to be a problem. At one point, I found that the clerk was allowing patients to schedule medication appointments in the middle of group therapy and to get such appointments with the internist without seeing me for an evaluation. Even our nurse was telling patients they had to go to group to get pills—not go to group to learn to manage their pain, depression, or life issues.

It was hard enough to convince the medical staff not to rely solely on medication for treatment. Without a policy consistently followed by all the staff and all the physicians in the clinic, addicts and others who didn't understand the importance of the whole program would have too much leeway to manipulate the system to get pills and not get the help that would make them better in the long run.

Even So, Some Addicts Got Better

Gloria Robbins was a forty-nine-year-old woman who had abused multiple drugs and alcohol for years. She had a third-grade education and had always been embarrassed about not being more successful. She had worked as a waitress on and off and traded sex for money when she could. She had pain and a number of medical problems and knew if she did not straighten out her life, she wouldn't be alive for long.

The first day I saw her, she had just been seen by the internist for the medical part of the evaluation. She was fuming when she came into my office. "That doctor thinks I'm faking to get drugs. I suppose you think the same thing. How am I to get any help around here if no one takes me seriously? I don't want any damn drugs. I had enough problems with that, but I need some help." She was much too angry to focus on anything I had to say, and although I mentioned that she could participate in one of our group sessions, I did not expect her to come back.

But come back she did, and she became one of the stars of the rehab group. She refused medications, embracing instead everything else offered her and in the process, turned her life around. You could see the pride in her expression at every step she took. Eventually, the social worker got Vocational Rehabilitation to agree to prepare her for the general educational development (GED) exam for high school equivalency, and she began to consider what job she might train for after that. Even though she might have qualified for disability based on addiction or various medical problems, she had another goal in mind. "I want to get an education and be somebody," she said to me one afternoon after the group. "No one ever believed in me before."

One advantage to working with addicts in a less-than-perfect program is that they have already learned how to live in a less-than-perfect world. They may have been abused themselves or live in a house where everyone is violent, uses drugs, steals, or is in and out of jail. Absorbing the imperfections of the medical system is just child's play by comparison. In fact, addicts can have great strength to overcome difficulty, given a little help and encouragement. Helping them to believe in themselves and find a direction for their energies is crucial in encouraging the change, as is the relationship with the doctor or medical team. Finding a passion in life other than drugs is the key.

CHAPTER NINETEEN

BUILDING THE ENDORPHIN
CLINIC PROGRAM

One of the first duties of the physician is to educate
the masses not to take medicine.
—Sir William Osler

Identifying Areas of Pain Prevention

Designing the Endorphin clinic was a golden opportunity to build a
program providing all the services that patients with chronic pain
and addiction would need, as well as to address some of the systemic
problems in the hospital that contributed to chronic pain in our patients.
That meant building a program that was not only patient-friendly, but
physician and hospital-friendly as well. So I looked for ways to save the
hospital money while providing better care for the patients.

Comprehensive and Timely Assessment

One way to accomplish this was to see patients when they wanted to
come in so there would be less need for emergency room visits or visits
to the general medical clinic. Another was to examine the patient and
refer those who needed specialty care: surgery to orthopedics, nerve
blocks to anesthesiology, and special treatment to neurology or rheu-
matology, while keeping the majority of chronic pain patients with
us. Our clinic would provide an in depth evaluation of all medical or

surgical conditions, physical, emotional, environmental factors, and the full range of rehabilitation services. That way the medical providers could treat as much or as little as they wanted with their patients, and leave general pain management and rehabilitation efforts to us.

Here is an example of one problem with the system as it was. After his insurance ran out, William George came to Cooper Green for surgery on a leg injury that kept him from working. By the time William came to see me for depression, he was eight months into a sixteen month wait for his first surgery appointment. During the eight months he had been waiting to see the surgeon, he had had no exercise or stretching program, and he was hurting more and more. The pain medicine was expensive, so he took as little of it as he could. I was horrified. With surgery, this man might have been walking again and able to return to work, but surgeons were so busy seeing non surgical patients who needed help with chronic pain, that they were unable to get him in for surgery in a timely fashion. William had not only become depressed, but by being inactive and inadequately treating his pain, he could increase his pain and make it chronic. We were able to treat his depression and get him moving again even though he still had to wait for the surgery. Eventually by seeing all patients first, we would be able to eliminate inappropriate referrals to surgery and send surgical candidates on without delays. This would be better for all patients, save money, and please the doctors in the specialty clinics who wanted to operate not pass out pills.

Medications are Part of the Evaluation

Early in the clinic planning, one of the ministers I worked with asked me to see his sister as a patient. She had been to pain clinics all over the east coast, but her pain was becoming worse. She had just returned from a month at a clinic in Philadelphia. I groaned inwardly, because the only place I was seeing patients for pain was at Cooper Green, and I did not have the full program up and running. I told the minister I would see his sister at Cooper Green, but I half expected she would not come.

A month passed, and one day, there was the sister in my pain treatment group. I explained that I usually saw people individually first, and that we would set up a time for her to come see me after group. Still, she participated gamely: "My name is Joann Waller. I'm a lawyer, but since I started having headaches, I can't work anymore." Though she listened intently to the other patients, I really did not expect her to come back after the first time, but there she was, week after week. Each time, she said something about herself and responded to the plight of others in the group.

After six weeks, her husband appeared in my office for an appointment. "Where is your wife?" I asked, surprised to see him there without her.

"She thought you might want to talk with me alone," he responded. The husband had brought Joann's previous treatment records; the pile was at least four inches thick. As he talked, I looked through them and saw that Joann had been in a number of programs stretching back five years. Several had been month-long residential pain programs, including the one in Philadelphia. She had had every test I knew about, and some I had never even heard of! Joan had been tried on every medication, and nothing seemed to make her any better.

"From what I can see, she's on a lot of medication," I said. "We may need to stop everything so we can see how much baseline pain she has. But let me look at these records and tell you what I think next time."

To my surprise, he stopped me. "Well, I don't know what you do at this clinic, but she's already better than she's been in a long time. She's not taking as much medication. And she even gets out and walks every morning, and she hasn't done that for several years." I knew from what Joann had said in group that her husband had insisted on sending her to one program after another, looking for answers. I couldn't help but wonder if this time, coming to Cooper Green had been her idea.

In the end she did have to be weaned off all the medicines before she got better. Medications have their place in the medical management of pain, but daily medication may make anyone worse. So, *everyone taking opiates regularly should get off completely, at least once a year,* for six weeks to two months. The same phenomenon may occur with other daily pain medication and additives like caffeine which causes rebound pain when they wear off. Beware! Mixing opiates with other pain medications, tranquilizers, sleeping pills, or alcohol can lead to serious difficulties, even death. Part of the medical rehabilitation involved careful evaluation of all drug interactions and side effects. Stopping opiates proved not to be practical with many patients until they became immersed in the rehabilitation program. Addiction issues would have to be considered eventually if the person could not give up the pills. Medication has its place in the treatment of pain, but daily medication can cause problems of its own and must be monitored closely.

The Endorphin Clinic Recovery Program

The recovery program developed in stages, but it was clear to me by the end that attending to all aspects of recovery was important for our patients. This involved not only correcting medial conditions and structural problems that could be addressed by surgery, working with medication, but addressing physical, emotional, social, occupational and spiritual rehabilitation as well.

Physical Rehabilitation

Preventing the development of chronic pain from shortened stiff muscles and tendons is the goal of physical therapy after surgery. Mabel Jones was sent to me for depression. She had had surgery on her knee eight months before and was now in a wheelchair. When I explored with her what her surgery had been for and what physical therapy she had had after it, I learned she had never been to physical therapy. "I was going to go," she said, "but we didn't have any money right then, and I thought I would wait until I was better and could go back to work before exercising. Moving made me hurt more." After I talked with Mabel's relatives, I learned she had once been the mainstay of her family, but she had never gotten over the surgery; she just hurt more and more.

I could treat her depression, but getting Mabel going again now that she had been inactive for so long was the challenge. Physical therapy is crucial to the recovery process after surgery to regain function. Here was one problem I hoped would be solved in the new clinic.

One plan that occurred to us was to change the billing system, so that charges for physical therapy and the therapy groups became part of the overall charge for surgery or for coming to our outpatient clinic. That way, patients would not have to choose between medications and rehabilitation. Patients, like the doctors treating them, needed to be educated about what it took to get well. Patients too often still believe that medicine or surgery alone is enough. Physical therapy or physical activity is essential after surgery to regain function and not hurt.

Changing the billing system to make rehabilitation part of the cost of surgery or recovery from illness meant that the hospital administration would have to approach Medicare and Medicaid about the change, or bill rehabilitation the same for everyone. (It is illegal to bill the government one way for indigent patients and another way for other patients.) The change would have to work for everyone, or it would work for no one.

The Danger of Inactivity

Muscles tighten around an injury. Inactivity causes muscles to shorten. So, often, physical therapy or the retraining of muscles and tendons can go a long way toward eliminating pain or keeping it at bay. Even for those with joint pain (arthritis) or old injuries, a daily routine that includes stretching, strengthening, and aerobic activities is beneficial.

Many so-called alternative or complementary therapies address physical rehabilitation or the retraining of muscles. Some therapies have a long tradition in healing going back thousands of years. Yoga, tai chi, and qigong combine movement with breathing and meditation that enhances flexibility, balance, relaxation, and strength. More recent techniques like Rolfing, the Feldenkreis Method, and the Alexander Technique also improve muscular balance and function. These all address musculoskeletal and mental health improvements at the same time. Even massage therapy, which comes in a number of forms, decreases muscle tension and stiffness, relieves muscle spasms, improves flexibility, and promotes healing and relaxation.

In our clinic we added simple yoga or tai chi moves that our patients could easily do, to the exercises and stretches they got from physical therapy. Fortunately, once the patients experienced the difference in themselves, they wanted to do more. We also provided a home exercise routine that involved moving every muscle and stretching around every joint, daily. This routine used the body or objects around the house as weights. It built activities into the patient's daily routine so it would be easier to remember. Being fit does not depend on going to a gym, but it does depend on a commitment to regular movement.

Doctors need to encourage patients to *move and stretch around each joint every day.* Too often, they tell their patients to let the pain determine their activity, implying, "Don't move if you hurt." Of course, patients need to know that *overdoing* will result in so much pain that they will not want to do anything. That is just as true of physical therapy as it is of housework. Physical therapy for an athlete can be much more strenuous than for someone who has just been sitting all day. For the in-active patient, a small daily exercise routine—perhaps four times a day, increasing gradually each week—is recommended. For those having difficulty beginning, starting with one stretch or one leg lift a day and adding one more every day may overcome the inertia of doing nothing.

Pain Prevention Aimed at Diabetes and Obesity

Hazel Jones was a morbidly obese twenty-four year old woman who sought disability benefits because she hurt too much to work. She had tried working in a cafeteria, but the standing hurt her too much. Since stopping work, she had gained more weight and now had diabetes. When we talked in the group about exercise or losing weight, Hazel said, "That's not my problem. I hurt before I gained weight."

Fortunately, Rosa Mae Cole and other group members spoke up. "I used to have problems with my feet and knees, too," said Rosa Mae, "but once I started losing weight and moving around more, the pain got better. Lots of people in my family have diabetes, and I was scared that if I didn't do something to lose weight and walk, I'd get diabetes, too. I don't hurt anymore. I haven't got diabetes yet, and maybe I can avoid getting it, too." She stopped, thinking for a minute. "My auntie lost her leg to diabetes, and I didn't want that to happen to me."

Diabetes and obesity have overwhelmed the medical system. Both require treatment and behavioral changes *over years*, not weeks or months. Cooper Green had a large number of patients with diabetes, mostly type 2. Most were overweight and were destined to develop chronic pain from the extra load on their joints and nerve damage from the diabetes, if they had not done so already. Many patients with diabetes had *never even attended a class on diabetes* and thus had never learned about the diet they should follow.

By using the power of our groups for education and modeling, we planned to involve these patients with others from the Endorphin Clinic to address exercise and nutrition issues together. Using as role models other patients who had already discovered the benefits of exercise and weight loss made it easier to educate and encourage those who either did not know these changes would make them hurt less or were in denial about how much difference exercise and a different diet would make.

Watching others struggle and yet overcome their pain was inspiring to many in the group who had felt pessimistic about themselves and their situations. Mary Sue Hite was reluctant to do anything. She had gained so much weight that she was moving less and less. She hurt everywhere. The group eventually got around her resistance and convinced her to stretch and do just a few exercises four times every day.

Because of the potential volume of the diabetic population who needed intervention and the potential costs, we planned to coordinate our approach through groups led by patient-volunteers, with specialists in diabetes, nutrition, and exercise to assist them. Our plan was to use mindfulness meditation and group reinforcement and mentoring.

Addressing Self-Defeating Behavior

Smoking. obesity, inactivity, social withdrawal, and addictions are all behaviors that make pain worse. Finding a way to address these self-defeating behaviors becomes important to overall recovery and the return to life. We used the power of the groups to discourage self-defeating behavior, with special patient-led groups providing education and a structured program to make changes. To change habits, having voluntary structures like the groups as well as finding a substitute activity or passion become important.

Meditation assisted with pain management, but it also allowed patients to become more mindful of their behavior in other areas of their lives. Pain may be a powerful motivator for changing eating, exercise, and smoking patterns, but a structured program using goal setting and resetting encouraged patients to do more. Once patients found the benefit of changing their smoking, eating, and exercise habits, they could inspire others to make changes and reinforce their own progress at the same time. Having struggled myself with weight issues, I knew we all need help at times to change habits and put up a spirited resistance.

Self-Management Workshops

In addition to weekly groups and individual education sessions, one of the social workers put on a workshop every three months with other staff members, volunteers from the community, and patient-volunteers to introduce patients to the many activities that benefit someone with chronic pain. These offerings included information about physical training, relaxation, guided imagery, stress management, yoga, nutrition, music therapy and distraction in the form of art or mathematical puzzles.

Nutrition training is important for addressing more than weight issues. Some foods actually increase inflammation and increase pain, while others do the opposite: act like aspirin in the body and enhance well-being. Increasing the foods with nutritional benefits and decreasing those with toxic or addictive properties can result in tremendous health benefits. Patients with gout, rheumatoid arthritis, osteoarthritis, neuralgia and diabetes may see the most benefit from a dietary change. All patients were encouraged to experiment and keep a journal to see how food affected their pain and their craving for more food. They might omit a food such as gluten in grains (wheat, corn, oats, rye), or dairy, meat, citrus fruit, nightshade vegetables (tomatoes, potatoes, eggplants and peppers), omega 6 oils (corn, safflower, or sunflower oil), shrimp, eggs, malt, soy, nuts, especially peanuts, chocolate or preservatives such a nitrites in cured meats. Caffeine containing beverages, like coffee and tea, and medicines were also suspect in those with chronic or recurrent pain, but these need to be decreased slowly, not stopped abruptly, to avoid rebound pain.

We also emphasized the negative aspects of sugar in large quantities and other dangerous elements of the American diet, along with the benefits of certain fruits (blueberries, raspberries, cherries, pineapple, dried currants, dates, prunes), ginger, curry powder, paprika, clove, garlic, peppermint, licorice, onions, gherkins, herbal teas, fatty fish (omega-3-oils), and a vegetarian diet. (See Jean Carper, *Food, Your Miracle Medicine,* for more information.)

As part of the self-management workshops, in addition to relaxation, we taught distraction using a variety of activities that shift the focus away from the painful area. Patients were surprised at the benefit of focusing attention on something other than themselves and pleased to have something they could initiate on their own. Some preferred mathematical puzzles; others, some form of art—be it painting, drawing, sculpting, or ceramics. *The relief of pain may even carry over for hours after the distracting activity.* Any really absorbing activity helps. Passively watching television will not do it, and any activity that aggravates an old injury may make the pain worse, not better.

In the workshops, we taught the use of music for relaxation and inspiration at the same time. Patients were encouraged to use music to promote healing, expressiveness, relaxation, and spiritual awareness.

CHAPTER TWENTY

EMOTIONAL, SOCIAL AND OCCUPATIONAL REHABILITATION

The world is full of suffering. It is also full of overcoming.
—Helen Keller

Emotional rehabilitation addresses negative emotions that are a problem in someone's life, and encourages positive emotions that bring about healing and recovery. Negative emotions make pain worse. Usually these are fear or anxiety, grief, horror, anger, hate, revenge, and depression. While medications assist with some of these and are useful adjuncts to treatment, finding a way to express such emotions frees the individual to move on from trauma or loss and embrace feelings which lessen pain and suffering.

Emotional rehabilitation addresses negative emotions that are a problem in someone's life, and encourages positive emotions that bring about healing and recovery. Negative emotions make pain worse. Usually these are fear or anxiety, grief, horror, anger, hate, revenge, and depression. While medications assist with some of these and are useful adjuncts to treatment, finding a way to express such emotions frees the individual to move on from trauma or loss and embrace feelings which lessen pain and suffering.

Tanya Roberts was an angry woman. She saw slight everywhere she looked. Pain from diabetic neuropathy and depression brought her to the group, but her real problem was her attitude about life. She was so angry, I was not sure how I would get through to her. Her mode of living was revenge. She had a running feud with her neighbors that had ended in physical fights and the police being called on several occasions. She always had a new grievance when she came to group: someone had pushed ahead of her in line or failed to help her when she dropped something. I knew anything I might say to her would be a waste.

Carl Davis was an elderly man who had lost a kidney in a street fight. He was now on kidney dialysis to live. He was too frail to get a kidney transplant, but though he had had a hard life, he was never angry. Everyone in the group looked up to Carl and his wisdom. "I was angry once," he said, softly one day. "Got into all kinds of fights and other trouble. I hated white people, cops, even my sorry neighbors. All I wanted to do was get even with everybody. It was eating me up, so much hate." He shifted his position as we all waited for him to go on. "All that hate was making me sick and that ended me up in the hospital. That's where I saw all those sick kids. Little ones that never hurt anyone. What was I doing wasting my time on all the bums in the world. I was in the hospital a long time, so I started visiting the children and telling them stories. They're so quick to smile, laugh. It made me feel better too, in fact, I started feeling real good just having a purpose everyday other than focusing on myself." You could see Carl getting tired as he spoke. I prayed that Tanya could hear him. She was so caught up in hate I was not sure that she could, but there were others who had listened hard. What an important message.

Understanding The Recovery Process

One day a young man appeared in group. He had sustained an injury playing football and felt his life was over. The group talked a lot about recovery and what is involved. I realized listening to him that he had a long way to go before he could think of himself as having a future. With loss, one has to grieve, and when one is young it may be years before a sense of peace and purpose returns to one's life. "You never really get well, do you?" the young man asked in despair. "You just have to get used to hurting all the time. The doctor says I'll always hurt, just get used to it." I wanted to tell him there was hope but when one is so young and has been told you will never be well, I felt helpless to say anything that would blunt the sting of what he was thinking and feeling. I turned to the group since these were people struggling with these questions themselves. Whether he could hear what they had to say, I did not know, but it had to be inspiring to hear how very positive they all were. I knew from my experience as a patient and watching other patients that recovery does occur. Pain does not have to dominate one's life and certainly you do *not* have to hurt all the time, but one has to make changes and work at doing better in a variety of ways to make recovery possible. The journey is not easy, but there are delights along the way, and one does not have to do it alone.

In the clinic, we had patients at all stages of recovery. Those further along were an inspiration and comfort to those just beginning. Recovery is different from just learning to live with something. How could I show this young man that recovery is different from just coming to terms with limitations, weakness? We get one year at each age. The paradox of life is that unlike a flower that reaches perfection and withers, in a human life, there is strength and weakness at each age, just as there is strength and weakness in each personality type and in each life circumstance. We can never grow back an amputated limb, but we can return to full functioning and even be stronger in some ways than before. Chronic pain, anxiety, depression, addictions and other self-defeating behaviors may stand in the way, but these can all be addressed, and we can recover not only from our affliction, but from the human burdens that weigh us down: hate, envy, greed and fear.

Recovery has different stages. Shock and disbelief at the time of trauma is often followed by the expectation that doctors will be able to repair the damage, or at least have medicine to get rid of pain. Somewhere along the way, patients must grieve their losses so they can begin to see what they need to do for themselves. Too many patients get stuck thinking a doctor will fix things, and that there is nothing they can do to get better. Many get depressed when they continue to hurt and feel bad; some even become suicidal.

Resistance to change was one of the biggest challenges in our clinic. Education about what to expect helped some make changes; some needed the threat of serious medical consequences. Others benefitted from seeing the effect of change on others in the groups. The support and inspiration of others was very important for many. Building community was very powerful as a tool to diffuse negative emotions that are so destructive.

As soon as patients began to exercise and feel encouragement from others, perhaps meditating or doing progressive relaxation as well to manage their pain, they began to get back a sense of control over their lives. They were encouraged to *act* well, even if they did not always *feel* well, in order to train their brains to *be* well. Then, as they felt more like themselves, they were encouraged to be more active and involved until they reached out to help others. Our challenge in the clinic was to facilitate each of these steps.

Social and Behavioral Rehabilitation

Acting well seems to be the key to getting well in the long run. As one man who had struggled with alcoholism put it, "Fake it until you make it." It seems that if you act like someone with self-esteem, you enhance your self-esteem. If you act like an athlete, you will more nearly reach the goal of becoming one. And if you act like a depressed couch potato, you will be a depressed couch potato. So we encouraged patients to act well until they were able to get well. The mantra here is *act well to get well! Fake it till you make it! Don't avoid! Set goals!* Some aspects of recovery are taken for granted, and some we seem to forget: in order to *get* well, we have to *act* well first. Setting goals and taking one step at a time toward being well is essential to the process of recovery.

The brain is endlessly pliable and has the capacity for growth well into old age, *in spite of damage to the brain itself.* So we must not avoid reengaging in all aspects of life, however fearful we may feel. Furthermore, since human beings are basically lazy, getting into a situation where we are forced to act is often necessary. Those who are sick for a long time with illness, depression, or chronic pain may need a boost to set goals, not avoid being active, and reengage with others. The structure of group therapy is useful to many for this reason. It also provides a forum for learning to deal with anger constructively.

Lewis Robins got married after over ten years in a wheelchair (an auto accident had injured his spinal cord). He had been looked after for so long that he had difficulty seeing that his healthy partner had needs of her own. Group talk helped Lewis to see that sitting down with his wife to discuss problems, say, once a week, was better than launching into complaints just as she got home from work.

Occupational Rehabilitation

Perhaps our biggest challenge was how to get patients focused on recovery when they had to stay disabled to get disability checks. I could identify with the fear that accompanies not being certain that you can go on without financial help. I also knew that anxiety about being unable to take care of oneself leads to disability on its own, so we needed a special program if we were to offset the disability trap.

Vocational Rehabilitation Services agreed to provide job skills training for our patients, so that they could feel free to work part-time without losing their disability money. Supporting the patient's quest for disability payments put the therapist in a position to also encourage patients to be active and productive, so we put together programs to assist those looking for disability compensation. Seeing the importance to everyone of being productive, we were then able to encourage having projects or working part time to be truly useful.

At all stages of life, being productive in some way is part of feeling alive. This was especially so for those who felt they could do little to contribute anymore. I remember one older man who was becoming weaker and weaker. During our discussion in group one day he said, "I looked around for something I could still do," He dabbed a moist cheek. "I found I could still iron clothes. So I help out my granddaughter who has to work, and I even make a little money on the side." I had noticed how sharp this man always looked in contrast to me in my slightly scruffy clothes. But not everyone is as wise as this man, so we made an effort to encourage useful activity to give meaning to life.

One must not lose sight of hobbies like sewing, knitting, jewelry making, carpentry, and gardening—or group activities such as choirs, bands, plays, or politics—as ways to be productive. Other useful occupations include volunteer organizations or causes important to the individual. Internships, where people can learn new skills and industries, can also work, but may be fairly demanding.

CHAPTER TWENTY-ONE

SPIRITUAL REHABILITATION

True happiness, we are told, consists in getting out of
one's self; but the point is not only to get out—you
must stay out; and to stay out you must have some absorbing errand.
—Henry James (from the novel *Roderick Hudson*)

Challenges of the Endorphin Clinic's Program

One challenge we faced was how to reinforce changes, not just over weeks or even months, but over years, in individuals who had trouble even paying the two dollars for parking. Addressing this was important for pain patients and those with diabetes and obesity as well. By using the power of the groups to train patients to help themselves and then help others, we thought we could expand indefinitely.

Patient-Volunteers

One of the most successful aspects of the program was the use of patient-volunteers. Patient-volunteers were those who had special skills or who had already mastered parts of the recovery program and had something to give back to others. Just as recovering alcoholics and addicts assist others in twelve-step programs, the idea was to match each patient with a sponsor—someone who was a little further along in the process—who could encourage the patient while reinforcing his or her own recovery at the same time.

The volunteers, with staff support and support from community volunteers with special skills, ran the ongoing groups devoted to exercise, nutrition, smoking cessation, and other issues. Together, these volunteers provided the nucleus for a motivational unit or team that would keep members on track and encourage them to share their own considerable survival skills. Because this was a volunteer program, there would be no charge to patients who participated, so they could attend as often as they wanted.

The patient-volunteer program proved to be very useful, most of all for the volunteers themselves. Tom Russell was a former college professor who, because of mental illness, had not been able to work for years. Although I tried to send those who were truly disabled for psychiatric reasons to the mental health centers, especially if I thought they might be suicidal, this man begged me to let him stay. "I've been kicked out of two mental health programs for not showing up," he said. "This is my last chance." Tom agreed that he would let me know if he was suicidal.

Tom would come to group weekly; then he would be gone for a month or two. I worried that he would kill himself eventually because he was so alone and was plagued by suicidal thoughts. At one point, he was so preoccupied with suicide that I arranged shock treatments and medication for him through the mental health center.

Often, Tom would come to group and say nothing. He might leave before his turn or stay just long enough to say his name. It was hard to tell if he was better. Once, I asked him what was helpful, and he said, "Here, I'm not pushed to do more than I can do." He felt a lot of guilt for letting his family down. He could not make himself call them on the phone. On those rare occasions that he went to family gatherings, he would bury himself in his room for weeks afterward, exhausted.

One day I realized I was going to be late for group the next week. I asked Tom if he could start the group for me. When I arrived, I could see he was doing well and gestured for him to continue. Running the group had an amazing effect on Tom. The group members who had worried so much about him were delighted to hear him speak up and participate. He spoke more than they had ever seen him do, and even talked a little about himself. It was interesting to see what he had learned from watching and listening to me over the years. His leadership was clearly good for him and for the others in the group. I asked him to lead the group with me on a regular basis.

The transformation in Tom was amazing. I had tried to find part-time volunteer work for him, thinking it would increase his self-esteem and help him be more active, but he could not find the initiative to start, even when he knew it would be good for him. Somehow, here, where he was known and where others were so delighted with his progress, he was able to open up more and more. His relationships with his children improved, and he was no longer plagued by suicidal thoughts.

After that, I added a few more volunteers when those with special skills or special needs appeared in the program. This was clearly beneficial to the volunteers and their own recovery process. At times, I asked who wanted to be a patient-volunteer. The idea that I thought they had something to offer meant a lot to some of patients, and some of the best volunteers were those with few natural skills who had overcome much adversity in their lives. The volunteers were helpful in designing parts of the program, filling in where they had special ability, and serving as mentors for those who were having more difficulty. Patient-volunteers were given training in co-counseling so they would have some skills helping other patients. The program gave volunteers a sense of self-worth and usefulness they had lost when they were hit with injury or illness, and it served as inspiration for those who had more work ahead of them.

Understanding Spiritual Rehabilitation

Though I had discovered the importance of connecting to something larger than myself in my forties as I recovered from pain and depression, it was only by watching my patients grow and get stronger that I began to fully appreciate what spiritual rehabilitation was all about. Sitting in group one Friday morning, I watched as those who had been suffering began to talk about what they were doing for others. Here were patients who had struggled with chronic illness, other losses, depression, and pain, finding a way to give to others. I was stunned. Here was surely the ultimate goal in the rehabilitation process: the capacity to give back and to care for others instead of staying focused on one's self.

One of the group members, Alfreda Martin, had come to me depressed and suicidal because she was about to lose her home and had no one in her life to help her. She had worked her whole life, cleaning at the hospital, but because of diabetes and heart disease, she couldn't continue. Still, she wasn't sick enough to get disability. She had one daughter who was ashamed that her mother had worked as a cleaner and didn't want to have anything to do with her.

Alfreda was so depressed that I was afraid she might end her life rather than face being homeless. Fortunately, she was able to use the support and love from the group members to help her through her despair and transfer to the Salvation Army shelter. One Friday morning, she appeared in the group looking like a foreign dignitary. Her robes were glorious and she had a turban on her head. Everyone marveled at the change in her. "They have lots of clothes and makeup at the Salvation Army." she said. "I've been putting clothes together for me and some of the others there. I didn't know how great it would make me feel to dress myself up. And others, too!" She found that her gift was to use donated clothes and makeup to make herself and others feel better. She had quite a flair.

Even after the Salvation Army found her a place where she could live on her own, she volunteered to help others at the shelter because she knew how hard it was to be homeless. Even as her health grew worse, she found more and more ways to reach out to others in need.

Another morning, Tony Salva came into group eager to tell how he had found ways to help his farm neighbors. Having sustained a severe injury to his left leg, he thought his days at the farm were numbered. But with regular exercise, he found he could do more than he had originally thought he would be able to. Now by driving his tractor, he could help his neighbors as well. He was ecstatic. "I thought all I'd have for the rest of my life was strong pills and having to be waited on by others. Being able to drive the tractor means I can do my part, and we can all work together to get the farm chores done."

Several weeks before, another group member had talked about his situation. Sam Phillips was a seventy-year-old man whose many medical problems and considerable pain made him very dependent on others. Sam had found that the group meetings and relaxation exercises we taught him helped a lot. He had been an alcoholic in youth, which had gotten him into one scrape after another, but he had settled down in his middle years and worked as a cook. Even as he had become too sick to work, he volunteered his services to cook for special events. Now, even though he could no longer cook even one meal, friends and acquaintances gathered to help him put on the parties for children and others that he was unable to do himself. Over and over, as people became involved and were able to move away from self-pity and self-focus, one could see them move to help others. This brought them out of themselves and made them part of the community. It made them smile and brought joy and delight back to their lives.

Sitting there in group that Friday morning, I had the sense of being in the most Christian community I had ever witnessed. I realized, watching these individuals from very diverse backgrounds responding to one another, sharing what little they had, that *empathy and the ability to love* constitute the ultimate human achievement, as well as the essence of Christianity and other great religions, however much fear and hate tend to derail the message of love.

How much suffering is needed to develop the capacity for empathy, love, and the ability to put the other first is uncertain, but hurting helps. It's true that hurting destroys some people, as can be seen in some survivors of concentration camps and other horrendous situations. But hurting offers others the opportunity to grasp ultimate truths about being alive. Even if one has wasted one's life hating others or pursuing wealth, hurting may be a wake-up call.

I had heard survivors of the German concentration camps speak of realizing things about life they could only have learned going through the horror of that experience. Here in the group, in the midst of people with difficult lives, I witnessed playfulness, joy, laughter, and endless creativity and love. They were like the Jewish survivors dancing in the streets, singing "L'chaim!" ("To life!"). Surely, this is the essence of being human.

Leaving Cooper Green

As I finished my time at Cooper Green, I could not help but think that having to work within the flawed complex inner workings of a hospital presents a great challenge, particularly when one is attempting to instill and encourage new concepts and methods. In spite of it all, patients are resilient, and even the poorest and most feeble have an amazing capacity to make the best of what is offered. All they need is to be recognized as the worthwhile human beings they are. I was privileged to have the opportunity to do that.

CHAPTER TWENTY-TWO

THE FIFTH VITAL SIGN

> Modern medicine is a negation of health. It isn't orga-
> nized to serve humans, but only itself, as an institution.
> It makes more people sick than it heals.
> —Aleksandr Solzhenitsyn

A mong the unfortunate steps medicine took to improve care for those in pain was the designation of pain as the fifth vital sign.[36] In 1995, the American Pain Society raised awareness of the inadequate care of those in pain, and in 1999, the Veterans Health Administration initiated a ten-point scale to measure pain as the fifth vital sign,[37] an idea that rapidly spread all over the country. That means that every time anyone measures a pulse or blood pressure, a pain level is sought. A question about pain might suggest that the nurse had an interest in whether the patient hurt, but in practice, it meant he or she needs a number to put on the chart.

The original idea was that an answer of above four out of ten on the pain scale would trigger a comprehensive pain assessment and rapid intervention by the nurses. But follow-up studies have shown that there has been no improvement in pain assessment or care for those in serious

---

36 The four traditional vital signs are pulse, respiration, temperature, and blood pressure.

37 Kirsch, H. Berdine, D. Zablotsky, et al., "Management Strategy: Identifying the Fifth Vital Sign." *Veterans Health System Journal* (2000) 149–159.

need of pain management, and that the focus on pain has instead led to an explosion of opiate prescriptions, increased addiction (with prescriptions being the main source of the drugs), and opiate overdoses and deaths.

The trouble is that pain is not something that can be measured in a trivial way. First of all, some people report a big number, and others a small one, yet there may not be a great difference in their actual levels of discomfort. The level of pain we report depends on how intent we are on the discomfort at a particular moment. Those who are anxious about hurting may report more pain than those who have acclimated to the discomfort (perhaps distracting themselves by writing poetry in their heads or focusing attention on some activity).

Pain assessment, which the pain scale was designed to trigger, has taken a back seat to addressing pain with pills. Assessing pain means checking whether the *causes of pain* are being adequately treated, including the part played by inactivity. Failure to stretch (or to do the right stretches), and failure to move even a little can make pain worse. Emotional factors need to be considered, as depression and anxiety worsen pain or may bring it on all by themselves. Social and occupational factors, plus addiction issues, are all potential causes of pain. Maybe opiates are aggravating the pain and need to be withdrawn or rotated with another opiate. All of this comes on top of assessing whether the tumor is expanding or has infiltrated the bone or the liver. or determining whether infection has set in or spread. All of these factors need to be looked at when a patient reports four or above on the pain scale, and appropriate intervention taken, but rarely does that happen because although the committee that proposed the intervention saw a benefit to their measurement, not all personnel charged with asking everyone their pain level is similarly committed to such a course. Of course they may be some limited places where this scale has been useful, but studies do not bear this out.

In addition, attention to pain without a comprehensive approach to assessment and targeted treatment, may lead to too much medication for pain and actually make matters worse. Also, getting the patient to focus on the pain may be counterproductive as attention tends to make pain worse. And repeated asking may make patients more anxious about hurting! Asking about pain has not only led to more prescriptions for opiates, it has put the emphasis on the wrong thing. If the medical establishment routinely asked about daily exercise and stretching, intake of fresh fruits and vegetables, changes in sleep patterns, or loss of interest in usual pursuits, doctors would have a measure that could indicate useful interventions and at the same time reinforce needed changes in the patient's daily routine. Focusing on pain *without investigating the underlying details,* has created a monster. Caveat emptor.

Certainly, the original intent of the American Pain Society and the Veterans Health Administration was to relieve suffering from severe pain and focus the doctor's attention on medical conditions needing additional care. It was based on the assumption that the doctor was not attending to new conditions that needed to be addressed, and that knowing how much the patient hurt would assist in that quest. What the exercise revealed instead is that doctors think the answer to more pain is more opiate medication. But even bone cancer patients whose pain worsens as the tumor expands, need assessment for everything that may be contributing to their pain. That way treatment can be focused to maximize their comfort without putting them at risk for more opiate side effects. Depression and anxiety can be addressed with stimulant medication which will make the opiate more effective and make the patient feel better and more alert. Inactivity may lead to tight, painful muscles that can be relieved by massage or a little movement and stretching in the bed. Increased pain at night may be related to tight muscles or to sleeplessness. Meditation, hypnosis, relaxation, and devices that manage muscle tension and pain can give the patient some control over discomfort, as can involvement in activities such as drawing, sudoku, and other distractions. Doctors must never forget that opiates themselves can worsen pain.

But I think a reassessment of making pain the fifth vital sign is in order. Hospice programs, cancer treatment centers, burn centers and other trauma centers may need special protocols to fit their patient's needs, but bringing this pain measurement into every physician's dealings with

every patient leads to mischief. While increasing routine nursing requirements does not automatically make for better patient care.

Opiate Use and Addiction Out of Control

Old ideas and prejudices, and not what we know from scientific studies
or even cultural wisdom, dominate the national discussion about opiate
use and addiction. The exponential rise in opiate and addiction problems
since I began writing this book shows me that the medical profession
must tackle the subject as soon as possible. It urgently needs to understand how best to use the full range of treatment options in all patients
struggling with chronic pain, depression, and chronic illness, but also to
reconsider how to manage opiates only to increase function while mini-
mizing the risks of toxicity, overdose and addiction. It urgently needs to
understand that human beings use substances, and substances are a great
boon to the practice of medicine, but this current spate of prescribing is
driven by cultural imperatives not in the best interest of the patient.

PHYSICIANS, HEAL THYSELVES!

CHAPTER TWENTY-THREE

DOCTORS ARE NOT GETTING THE WORD

What happens then is like what happens when we sepa-
rate a jigsaw puzzle into its five hundred pieces; the
over-all picture disappears. This is the state of modern
medicine: It has lost the sense of the unity of man. Such
is the price it has paid for its scientific progress. It has
sacrificed art to science.
Paul Tournier, MD

Medicine is of all the Arts the most noble; but owing
to the ignorance of those who practice it, and of those
who, inconsiderately, form a judgment of them, it is at
present behind all the Arts.
—Hippocrates

As a young person during the Vietnam War, I had already lost my belief in authority figures well before I became a psychiatrist. Growing up in a navy family, I could see that people in positions of power could be wrong. Still, as a resident in psychiatry in 1976, I looked forward to hearing all the experts at my first psychiatric meeting, the World Congress for Psychiatry in Honolulu, Hawaii.

Beautiful as Hawaii was, I was so fascinated with the sessions that I went from one to another, from morning to night. I heard the biological psychiatrists with their amazing new medications, the psychoanalysts who addressed major hang-ups, the family therapists who healed relationships, the experts on trans-sexualism, and more. I went to each new offering thrilled with the delight of discovery. Even the political meetings were interesting as the World Congress voted to censure the Russians for using psychiatric hospitals for political purposes and for diagnosing dissidents as mentally ill. In fact, I was so enthralled that on my very last morning there, instead of heading for the beach I went to the last conference on the program, one put on by the Organization of Orthomolecular Psychiatrists.[38]

At that time, the orthomolecular psychiatrists were held in disrepute by many in the profession. These orthomolecular psychiatrists claimed that their program, which included mega-doses of vitamins, helped patients with schizophrenia.[39] The psychiatric community apparently felt that it was the psychotropic medications leading to improvement, not the other interventions.

I went to this meeting out of curiosity, expecting to see a bunch of charlatans. I found instead a group of extremely knowledgeable physicians—who were the *only ones during the whole week who acknowledged all the advances in psychiatry and used all of them with their patients.*

By employing all these advances, including vitamins and nutrition, they needed *less* medication to control patients' psychotic symptoms. Since they prescribed less medicine, their patients experienced fewer side effects and were more apt to keep taking the medicine. Since they also involved the patients' families and considered their relationships and other concerns, these doctors promoted stability in their patients' lives and reduced the stress that might set off a new round of psychotic symptoms or dangerous behavior.

Hearing all of this, I was shocked. Wow! How could it be that these psychiatrists, reviled by the profession, were the only ones who knew what they were doing? How could all the experts in each field fail to

---

[38] The term "orthomolecular" was coined by Dr. Linus Pauling in 1968 to describe the investigation into natural causes and treatments.

[39] Linus Pauling, "Orthomolecular Psychiatry," *Science, New Series* 160 (3825) (April 19, 1968): 265–271.

acknowledge the advances in all the other fields? After this experience, I became skeptical of new gurus and trends in psychiatry. I did not trust anything unless I could check it out myself or it conformed to my own experience.

Advances in medication have revolutionized psychiatric treatment, yet individuals with schizophrenia are living on the street, using disability money to buy street drugs that set off more psychosis until they get readmitted to the hospital, re-medicated, and sent out again. Without the support that gives them a chance to live a more stable life, they just get stuck in a revolving door—an example of individual freedom gone amok. Psychotherapy's many forms—individual, group or family therapy, along with nutrition, exercise, and physical well-being—are valuable in the treatment of psychiatric illness, but these methods are no longer championed by the profession. Everything today seems to boil down to brain chemistry and pills. To understand how such a travesty takes place, one only has to look at psychiatry's recent history.

In the nineteenth century, Freud became interested in the problems of patients who exhibited chronic physical symptoms that were unresponsive to all treatment. In an attempt to scientifically quantify and qualify the origin of these symptoms, Freud separated unconscious from conscious mental processes. He determined that there were interacting conscious and unconscious mental mechanisms for responding to pain, pleasure, and anxiety.

Further, he observed issues in the doctor-patient relationship that could affect the treatment of these conditions. In particular, he described *transference*, the shifting of the patient's feelings from previous relationships onto the doctor, so-called projection, and *countertransference*, the doctor's shifting of feelings about others onto the patient. He believed that these reactions determined the success or failure of the doctor-patient relationship. Freud meticulously and forthrightly described what he observed; and while he was limited by the ignorance of his time, he opened the door to our understandings of the interactions of the mind and emotion with the body. His work demonstrated the value of understanding the relationship between physical symptoms and emotional and personality issues. It also demonstrated how and why no doctor is able to be completely neutral.

World War I soldiers afflicted with shell shock and extreme emotional reactions to war spurred physicians' interest in the mind-body connection. Drs. Franz Alexander and Felix Deutsch led the field.[40] Around 1922, Deutsch called the emerging study of how emotional factors affected illness *psychosomatic medicine,* and in 1939 the *Journal of Psychosomatic Medicine* was created to disseminate its research. More psychiatrists began to work in medical settings, especially after World War II; they were interested in medical and surgical patients who showed emotional reactions to illness or hospitalization, the trauma of disease, or the trauma of a surgical experience such as amputation. Physicians also began to recognize failures and compromises in the doctor-patient relationship that affected treatment and, ultimately, outcome.[41]

In 1956, Dr. Grete Bibring, a Viennese psychoanalyst and the first female professor at Harvard Medical School, published her seminal paper underscoring the inseparability of the mind and body and the importance of "personality diagnosis" in history taking and case formulation for all patients. Bibring wrote, *"In the doctor's work, psychological understanding is of profound importance. It evokes in the patient all his positive strength, his willingness to cooperate, and his constructive wish to get well and do right by himself and by his doctor. Thus, the optimal psychosomatic condition is established that may make the difference between a patient who wants to live and the apathy and sabotage of the patient who lets himself die."*[42]

In the 1950s, physicians considered certain illnesses psychosomatic—that is, brought on by emotion—but others not. Today,

---

[40] Felix Deutsch, "Psychoanalysis and Internal Medicine" (1927), in Franz Alexander, et al., eds. *Psychoanalytic Pioneers* (Transaction Publishers, 1995).

[41] Brand, *The Gift Nobody Wants.*

[42] Grete L. Bibring, The Grete L. (Grete Lehner) Bibring Papers, 1882-1977, H MS c159. Harvard Medical Library, Francis A. Countway Library of Medicine, Boston, MA

even as practicing physicians focus more on medication and technology, we know that emotions and the doctor-patient relationship affect the course of *all* illnesses, as well as recovery from injury or surgery. Psychosomatic research has increasingly emphasized multi-causality in illness. Conflict and stress have many causes that impact the health of the individual. They include job loss, disturbed family relationships, the loss of important figures in one's life, separation, bereavement, difficult doctor-patient relationships, feelings of helplessness and hopelessness, grief on the anniversary of a loss, and emotional aspects of illnesses that are life-threatening or are likely to result in disability. In the end, it may be one's personality that determines his or her response to these adversities. Character matters. Grit matters.

Bio-psycho-social Model of Psychiatry

After World War II, Dr John Bonica, an anesthesiologist, began taking an interest in those patients who did not respond to standard medical treatment. To address the problem he was seeing he sought the help of specialists in psychiatry, psychology, physical medicine, and others. From this grew the multi-disciplinary pain movement.

At the same time as the new pain clinics were opening, 1964, psychiatrist George Engel initiated the bio-psycho-social model of psychiatry as a blueprint for research, a framework for teaching, and a design for action in the real world of health care. He pointed out that the traditional medical model left no room for the social, psychological, and behavioral dimensions of illness. By focusing on only the biomedical aspects of disease, it limited what was available to help patients get better. He studied chronic pain and the psychological adaptation to illness.[43] Both psychiatry and medical practice seemed to be moving to bring together all avenues to treat chronic pain.

---

[43] George Engel, "The Need for a New Medical Model: A Challenge for Biomedicine," *Science* 196 (1977): 129–136.

Still, Doctors Are Not Getting the Word:
Problems in Psychiatry

We now know much about pain and how the mind interacts with the body to bring about healing, but American doctors are not being taught this information. One of the main reasons for this failure is the splintering of factions in psychiatry. The Psychosomatic Association, consultation-liaison groups, the many pain associations, biological psychiatry groups, and psychoanalytic groups all do research, but they mainly talk among themselves, not to one another. Another problem has been the divisions within the profession between the American Psychiatric Association (with its consultation-liaison division, or general hospital psychiatry) and the American Psychosomatic Association. Since 2003, the Academy of Psychosomatic Research has been trying to pull together disparate groups in this field, but there are still many organizations addressing chronic pain and its issues in only limited ways.

Although medical educators came to agree that psychiatric training would be important for all medical students since an understanding of the mind-body connection was important for all physicians, the training was often not performed by those knowledgeable about psychosomatic issues.

Most psychiatric training programs and the psychiatrists they produce are biologically oriented; that is, they are not trained in psychosomatic medicine, psychological or behavioral medicine, or even the importance of the doctor-patient relationship. They remain focused on the biomedical aspects of psychiatry and not on the psychodynamic aspects of the profession. In addition, practitioners in departments of psychiatry must see patients with major mental illnesses like schizophrenia, and most medical students take part in these programs rather than being in contact with psychiatrists who treat medical and surgical patients with depression, anxiety, pain and delirium. This means the student may not be exposed to the right concepts.

The medical world, increasingly dominated by cost-based programs has increased pressure on psychiatrists to focus on medication at the expense of psychotherapy. The fact that most medical practitioners use psychologists rather than psychiatrists to work with their patients has not helped. Psychologists are often better trained in psychodynamic and relationship matters while psychiatrists have moved to the physical and biological realms. Many psychologists are trained as behaviorists—to see all behavior as a result of conditioning. The battles between psychology and psychiatry over areas of practice and the ability to prescribe medications foster conflict rather than collaboration. Rather than see that each has something to offer, psychiatrists and psychologists have become adversaries who compete for different parts of the market.

In addition, a coordinated mind-body education for physicians has been difficult to develop, because even psychiatrists can not agree about the ways the body and mind interrelate. One example is the physical symptoms that have gone unrecognized in patients suffering from depression, while another is the psychiatric research that persistently searches for psychogenic or emotion based pains. Separating the emotional from the *real* physical pain problem is always elusive, but many still believe in trying. In fact, there is no solid evidence for allegedly psychopathological pains being any different from so-called *real* physical pains, as Valerie Hardcastle demonstrates in *The Myth of Pain.*[44] *All pain is based in emotion.*

At this rate no one person (or even specialty) can absorb all new discoveries or advances in all areas relevant to a field of practice at the current rate of publishing, much less sort out all the nonsense promoted by various factions. In his book *Harmony of Illusions*, Allen Young points out that even a scientific study can be incorrect.[45] He chronicles how a host of methodological and conceptual problems recurrently emerges to distort information gleaned from studies.

In addition, the holistic health movement, the emergent mind-body medicine, and Norman Vincent Peale's and Norman Cousins's *positive thinking* movement, all popularized the power of suggestion and

---

[44] Valerie Gray Hardcastle, *The Myth of Pain* (Cambridge: MIT Press, 1999), 21.
[45] Allan Young, *The Harmony of Illusions: Inventing Post-Traumatic Stress Disorder* (Princeton, NJ: Princeton University Press, 1995)

the placebo effect. Is it any wonder that confusion reigns? The good news is that these ideas are all out there in the culture somewhere, so that even if they are not in vogue in medical practice at the moment, they are not lost.

The Role of Organized Medicine

Over the years organized medicine has sought to define what is standard medical practice, weeding out those whose activities may harm patients. Even in the eighteenth century, organized medicine pushed for the regulation of irregular healers, even when there was evidence that magicians, charlatans, and quacks could bring about powerful healing.[46]

In late eighteenth-century Paris, Anton Mesmer claimed to have powers to heal. People would come from far and wide to touch the hem of his robe. When there were too many, he held out a long rod to allow many more to be in contact with him. With this he cured hundreds of suffers, even some in too much pain to walk. His charisma became so powerful that he could merely will the pain away (a practice long used by shamans and other early healers). But the scientific community rejected him and accused him of being a charlatan. Mesmer left Paris and died in disgrace. Today, we call his gift mesmerism or hypnosis.

In modern times we have come to regard magicians, charlatans, and quacks with suspicion, but we in the medical profession may have to rethink the role of healers and what is involved in the process of healing.

---

[46] Barbara B. Schnorrenberg and O. M. Brack, Jr., eds., "Medical Men of Bath," vol. 13 of *Studies of Eighteenth-Century Culture*, American Society for Eighteenth Century Studies (Madison, Wisconsin: University of Wisconsin Press, 1984).

CHAPTER TWENTY-FOUR

THE DOCTOR'S INFLUENCE ON SELF-DEFEATING BEHAVIOR

The good physician treats the disease; the great physician treats the patient who has the disease.
—William Osler, MD

It is highly significant, and indeed almost a rule, that moral courage has its source in identification thorough one's own sensitivity with the suffering of one's fellow human beings.
—Rollo May

A major challenge in treating any long term illness is managing self-defeating behavior. A self-defeating behavior may be anything from failing to follow the doctor's orders, to eating the wrong food, smoking or drinking too much, lashing out with anger, or failing to exercise and stretch regularly. While many factors determine which self-defeating behaviors are most important in the course of any particular medical illness, patients who do the right things to take care of themselves do better than those who do not. The doctor's interventions may be crucial in making this happen, but that means assessing the patients strengths and weaknesses, understanding where the patient needs information, structure or support, and dealing with the patient's emotions.

This may mean overcoming the patient's initial anger and refusal to cooperate with treatment or change—working through resistance when it first appears and when it reemerges in the course of treatment. If the physician or the treatment team react negatively and defensively to the patient's resistance or negativity, this will only make the patient more stubborn and compound the problem.

Motivation is key to a patient's recovery from chronic pain and chronic illness. Motivation to recover—even to live—may be lacking when a patient faces depression as a result of overwhelming stress, illness, or pain. The doctor-patient relationship can and docs play a major role in bolstering resolve until the patient is able to motivate him- or herself. Even the act of giving a prescription, a handout, or medication samples may represent the tangible support needed to get the patient through.

Beneficial doctor-patient relationships are based on the willingness not only to advise, but to *listen* to the patient. And doctors must listen to the words as well as the nonverbal expressions and the meaning behind the words. This involves empathy, or the ability to see things from another's point of view. Doctors are so accustomed to looking at things from the scientific point of view that they often have difficulty shifting gears and seeing what is important in the patient's eyes.

Empathy: Really Listening

The best example I ever heard of empathy is a story told in the book *Emotional Intelligence* by Daniel Goldman. The story goes more or less like this. A strong, caring man just returning from a karate lesson encounters a belligerent drunk on the subway. The storyteller is trying to decide when to tackle this dangerous man to protect others from the perceived threat. While he is debating what to do, another man, smaller and older, sits down next to the drunk, takes out his lunch, and offers some to the agitated man. "You must be tired," he says. "Sit down and share my sandwich with me." Then, after a pause, he says, "You look like you've had a hard day. Why don't you come home with me and get a good hot meal? My wife isn't the best cook, but she can be depended on. Do you have family?"

At this point, the drunk bursts into tears. "My wife says she can't take it anymore. She went home to Kansas. My life is over without her." He sobs into his hands, and suddenly, the danger is past.[47]

It's really the same with patients. It's only in really listening to verbal and nonverbal communications that doctors can begin to tease out small parts of the personal story so they can *get at the real feeling* behind the belligerence, the silence, the hysterical symptom, or whatever else is relevant to the moment. And it doesn't even matter if all the kind guesses aren't right! People can sense the genuineness behind the doctor's words, and respond to that. This allows the sufferer to get to the bottom of the fears, uncertainties, or loss and puts him or her in a position to work out problems without the interference of his own defensive maneuvers.

What is so powerful about the story of the drunk man and the reactions of those around him is that it demonstrates what is most important in dealing with other human beings: empathy. Generally, our idea of the ultimate in human heroism and sacrifice is taking on and fighting a dangerous person, organization, or nation. We even see it as a sign of weakness to try to see what things look like from the other person's point of view. But that's exactly empathy is—walking in another's shoes.

Empathy: The Ultimate Goal of Spirituality

Empathy is the major objective of all of the great religions (although the resurgence of fear and violence obscures it from time to time). Seeing things from someone else's point of view is the ultimate human achievement and the ultimate goal in the recovery process. I don't think that "turn the other cheek" means to stand there and let yourself be beaten; it means turning your head so you can listen to another's concerns and point of view. It means to really listen, not from the narcissistic, self-protective position we see too often in the world today, but from the position of understanding.

---

[47] Daniel Goleman, *Emotional Intelligence: Why It Can Matter More Than IQ* (New York: Bantam Books, 1995).

Difficult People Look Like They Have Personality Disorders

Any patient who is depressed or in pain, an addict or not, may appear to have a personality disorder. In fact, one study showed 62 percent of patients diagnosed with borderline personality disorder actually suffer from chronic pain syndromes, while 60 percent of chronic pain patients have a diagnosed personality disorder.[48] Sansone and Associates identified features of borderline personality disorder in 47 percent of patients with chronic pain who attended a family practice clinic and noted that "staff members need to be informed about the diagnosis of personality disorder to avoid reinforcing the patient's inappropriate or manipulative behavior."[49]

Dr. George Vaillant has pointed out that a diagnosis of borderline personality disorder is more likely to be made when the examiner does not like the patient.[50] Thus, the demanding, threatening, manipulative patient is more likely to be given such a diagnosis. That is why seeing things from the patient's perspective is the only effective way to understand his or her behavior.

Prejudging Patient Behavior

I saw a stunning example of the misjudgment of a patient in my senior year as a psychiatric resident. I was on call for hospital admissions when I heard from the staff that a new patient was the *worst patient they had ever seen.* On a previous admission, Mrs. Sara Gage had been labeled with a diagnosis of borderline personality disorder under stress. Her chart indicated that she had been a problem on the unit throughout her hospital stay. Now she was about to be readmitted, and the whole staff

---

[48] Dawn A. Marcus, "Tips for Managing Chronic Pain: Implementing the Latest Guidelines," *Postgraduate Medicine* 113, no. 4 (April 2003).

[49] Randy A. Sansone and Lori A. Sansone, "Review: Borderline Personality and the Pain Paradox," *Psychiatry MMC* 4(4) (2007): 40–46.

[50] George E. Vaillant, ed., *Empirical Studies of Ego Mechanisms of Defense* (Washington: American Psychiatric Press, 1986).

reacted even before she arrived. When I first saw her, Mrs. Gage was so agitated that four people had to carry her in and restrain her. The nurses wanted me to sedate her immediately.

The staff's hostility made me uncomfortable, so I went in to see if I could talk with Mrs. Gage before I sedated her. "Mrs. Gage," I began, "I'm Dr. Carmichael. Do you think you can calm down enough so I can talk with you?" She nodded her head and said yes. I asked everyone else to leave the room and sat down. Agitated patients frequently calm down when no longer challenged.

The story Mrs. Gage told was this: A beauty queen at the age of eighteen, she had married her high-school sweetheart. Her husband had entered her father's business, and now, at age forty, he was president of the company. She had become a slightly dumpy middle-aged housewife. Life had been fine until her husband's twenty-two-year-old female assistant started taking business trips with him. Then, during sex with his wife, he foolishly started telling her of his sexual fantasies about this beautiful young assistant. At that point, Mrs. Gage went ballistic.

Once she finished her story, she felt understood. And once she understood we would have sessions with her husband she realized she was going to get the help she needed with him. From then on, she was no problem to the hospital staff. In fact, she became a model patient. She required no medication to control her behavior or otherwise. After some sessions with the husband, she was able to leave the hospital, ready to build a more mature relationship at home. Being understood put her in a position to work out her own problems with her husband.

Personality Disorder Labels Are a Reflection on the Labeler

Patients like Mrs. Gage who are under stress can appear to have personality disorders because their response to anger and stress can make them seem irrational. Furthermore, patients who are in pain, depressed, or under stress may resist doing what others want them to do. In medicine, we call that noncompliance. Such behavior may suggest a personality disorder to those who do not know any better. But noncompliance—not following doctors' orders—is more frequently a sign of depression that the doctor needs to explore. Personality disorder labels often represent the attitude of the labeler rather than tell us anything about the patient.

Depressed People Tend to Be Difficult

Depressed individuals may be difficult and unpleasant, lapsing into self-defeating behaviors that make them only more depressed. Giving the patient a personality disorder diagnosis, rather than identifying the source of the depression or stress and helping the person deal with the stress or loss, is counterproductive, even if it feels good to the professional frustrated with a difficult patient. Doctors deal with people who are under stress and facing loss constantly; giving such patients a personality disorder diagnosis may not only be inaccurate, but tends to prejudice the staff, which makes them less helpful.

Recognizing that the root problem is anger, not willfulness, allows the treatment team to explore the roots of the problem and be in a position to teach new behavior so a patient can act, think, and feel more successful. From there, setting small, doable goals and evaluating what works and what does not work can help patients through the initial phases of any behavioral change. But the medical staff must listen first before they react.

Behavior modification techniques are a popular feature in the *Diagnostic and Statistical Manual of Mental Disorders* (DSM-IV)[51]; they may be necessary for patients who use recurring and predictable manipulations to obtain addicting medications or who use suicide threats to gain hospital admission, but it is always safest to consider the way things look from the patient's point of view before initiating such measures. Too often, the application of behavior modification leads to a characterization of the patient that merely reflects a medical professional's bias or lack of training.

---

[51] DSM-5 coming out May 2013

The Structure of Modern Medicine Creates Problems

For the most part, modern medicine is not based on the patient's relationship with the doctor. Patients are expected to interact with nurses and other medical personnel and not bother the doctor. Failure to have a close tie to the doctor creates problems because physicians are human, and they react out of self-interest rather than the patient's interest if the patient is just a name on a chart. We are hard wired to respond to the needs of others, but we have to be in relationship with them to get that response.

As sociologist Marvin Harris points out in his book *Why Nothing Works*, the further the consumer is from the producer of a product, the less the producer cares about the consumer.[52] That is just as true in medicine as in other relationships. The more medicine is run like a business with emphasis on cost-effectiveness, the less likely doctors are to know their patients well enough to have a relationship.

Physicians Get Anxious, Too

Anxiety about being fooled often leads physicians to doubt patients. Once a doctor becomes anxious, he or she stops being a good listener and tends to operate from his or her own prejudices and assumptions. Rather than obtaining complete and accurate information from the patient about his or her irritability or anger, the doctor tends to react defensively. But when a physician is thoroughly trained to obtain specific and detailed information about a patient's behavior or expressed emotions, he or she is better able to deal with his own anxieties and not overreact to unexpected patient behaviors. Without such training, a doctor may cease to see that the patient is his best ally to help sort out what is going on.

Worse still, in today's litigious climate, the doctor may even see the patient as a potential threat. One physician told me that he saw every

---

[52] Marvin Harris, *Why Nothing Works: The Anthropology of Daily Life* (New York: Simon and Schuster, 1987), 17.

patient who came through the door as a potential adversary. How can anyone be empathetic under those circumstances? But today's fast-food medicine means that patients are primed to sue when something goes wrong. I remember in my youth doctors weeping with their patients and families when something went wrong. Can you imagine that happening today? Not only does the doctor have less of a chance to know this person he is treating, but the patient has less chance to see the physician struggle and care about him or her in return.

Can Empathy Be Taught?

Perhaps the real question is, can empathy be taught—and learned? Or is empathy something you are born with? My guess is that it's follows a one-third rule: one-third have it, one-third can develop it, and one-third will never get it, no matter what we do. Statistics on medical school admittees show that they are less empathetic than in the past.[53] What part of that is due to our increased tolerance for the violence and sadistic behavior witnessed nightly on our television screens and in movies, what part is due to less direct involvement with patients, and what part is due to the kind of people choosing to enter medicine today, is uncertain.

Robert L. Lifton did a study of the physicians in Germany responsible for inhumane medical experiments.[54] His findings were that those doctors weren't what we think of as monsters or psychopaths; they were just average, good-old-boy doctors who took their families to church on Sunday—*who did what they did to survive.* The capacity of ordinary people to do brutal things is well documented. We would like to think our doctors capable of a level of integrity beyond the ordinary, but in a country where medicine has become a road to success and money, empathy, and integrity along with it, may get short shrift. Integrity and empathy get even harder when patients look very different from the treating doctor: obviously poor, from another race or culture, and

---

[53] Robert Finn, "Study: Students Enter Medical School with 'Empathy Deficit.'" *Ob-Gyn News* (July 1, 2003).

[54] R.J. Lifton, *Home from the War* (USA: Harper Basic Books, 1973), 417.

especially when a patient is an addict. Even generally decent physicians in this country could mistreat those in a despised category, as we did to Japanese, Jew, black or conscientious objector in World War II.

It becomes all too easy to forget the human needs of the sick, the poor, and the very young or old when the focus in medical care is on business. This may be especially so in a society that refuses to protect the weak from gun violence, pornography and sadistic behavior on television, provide adequate nutrition and education for all the very young, or provide medical insurance that protects anyone in need instead of the for-profit medical providers and pharmaceutical companies; even under the Affordable Care Act. As we watch the co-optation of political power by moneyed interests, and pay lip service to individual rights rather than address our human responsibility to one another, when law becomes the standard of behavior, not what is right, just or fair; when doctors offer prepaid *concierge* medicine to solve the problem of too little time with patients; rather than speak up for those who are most in need, we are witnessing an erosion in medical standards in this country that threatens to rival the horrors of the past. We must recognize the signs now and not kid ourselves that because we provide the most sophisticated hi tech surgery available, that we are not lagging in too many other ways. Physicians have always fought for what was best for their patients and must find a way to do so again. Their souls depend on it.

But patients can help. When dealing with their own doctors, they can try to see things from the doctor's point of view and make empathic comments which bridge the relationship gap so well. I find if I want to doctor listen to me, I first listen hard to the doctor's concerns. This frees his mind to hear me and facilitates the connection between us that lets him listen to what I have to say. I am not sure how we became a nation where we look for someone to blame when things go wrong rather than take responsibility for finding a solution ourselves, the position of blame is an immature one, it may make us feel better, but it does not solve the problem ahead. Like revenge it eats at us and creates problems for the future.

FINAL
THOUGHTS

CHAPTER TWENTY-FIVE

AND THEY LIVED HAPPILY EVER AFTER

My barn having burned to the ground,
I can now see the moon.
—Masahide, Japanese poet

Blessings and Loss

Starting in the late nineties, I experienced firsthand that every relationship comes to an end. Friends, family, and mentors died. My
children grew up and moved into their own lives on different sides of
the world. My oldest friend took to the bottle and ended up among the
derelicts in New York City. I had already experienced divorce some
thirty years before. These losses provided sobering insight into how life
works. But then, good fortune smiled on me. At sixty-one, I fell in love
with a wonderful man who loves me, too.

Looking back, I recognize that good fortune has smiled on me in
many ways. I made it to my late sixties still practicing medicine in an
area I found rewarding and important, and after I retired, I have written the book (actually, two) that I had wanted to write for at least thirty
years. Beyond that, I have survived multiple sclerosis without having
to take any of the routinely prescribed medicines. I just had to shake
my head two years ago, when I sought the help of another specialist
in multiple sclerosis to see if it would be safe for me to take a flu shot
after all these years. After reviewing my information, he told me that
after forty-three years, *"You must have relapsing remitting multiple*

sclerosis"—(That is, the best kind.)—*"only it didn't remit!"* (That is, it did not go away.)

Multiple sclerosis has taken a toll on my energy. Planning ahead allows me to do more, but many times, I have felt I just could not go on working and recovering, day after day. One particularly difficult year, I chanced upon a book by George Leonard called *Mastery*. An expert in the martial art of aikido, Leonard writes about the importance of mastering the things we do in our day to day lives, not just living for the peak moments of winning or success. As someone who struggled with pain and partially paralyzed muscles, I knew that for me life could no longer center around being the best or winning; but until I read Leonard, I had seen being less than the best as a failure. Growing up in America, competing in sports, academics, even socially, I had always been able to win. Now this book opened my eyes to the idea that the real success in life was in the mastery of its every aspect of that life: our relationships, our jobs, our hobbies, and even our physical bodies.[55] The key was being able to enjoy mastering each challenge, each plateau or stage along the way. I had mastered the pain in my life by religiously stretching and exercising, enjoying many steps along that path, and I now found it possible to master other areas of my life, even though they seemed just as daunting at times, including writing this book.

Inspired by Leonard's philosophy, I looked for a training program near home that would teach a disciplined approach to mastery. What I found was John Bright-Fey's Blue Dragon Academy, which used tai chi, kung fu, and aspects of other eastern disciplines to train the body and the mind. I attended classes for a couple of years. I could not leap or do some of the other feats, but I noticed that it no longer bothered me. I knew that my true goal was to enjoy the process of mastering each step that I *could do*. After class I noticed that I had more energy to do other things in my life. Before taking the class I had trouble getting myself to get up and go swimming in the morning. After taking the

---

[55] George Leonard, *Mastery: The Key to Success and Long-Term Fulfillment* (New York: Plume, 1992).

class, it became easy to get up. Rather than feel overwhelmed by my responsibilities, I once more had the energy to go on.

Later, I found John Bright-Fey's book, *A Morning Cup of Tai Chi*,[56] which enabled me to develop my own morning routine at home. In conjunction with aerobic exercise, a routine of movement, stretching, and breathing that works out stiffness, improves balance, and focuses the mind helps me continue the gradual process of improvement, whatever my level of strength or flexibility at the moment. Further, focusing on what I *can* accomplish facilitates continual recovery and enhances self-esteem

Lessons of a Lifetime

I know I began absorbing lessons about pain at an early age. Both my mother and grandmother were great models for living well with pain.

My grandmother was knocked off the sidewalk in her sixties, breaking her hip. Hip replacement surgery came along when she was ninety, but the doctors told her she was too old for the surgery. At ninety-five she said she would take the risk and have the surgery. She had to lie flat for three months after surgery before they would let her sit up. During that time she wrote poems in her head to keep herself focused, and perhaps distract herself from focusing on the pain following surgery. In one poem, she quoted from the sundial: "Count Only Sunny Hours." That was her credo. She lived to a hundred and three and a half and wrote her memoirs after her hundredth birthday. She sat at an old-fashioned typewriter in her bedroom, looking as beautiful as a porcelain doll with her skin as white as alabaster. Since she was mostly blind by then, she stuck corn plasters to the typewriter keys so her fingers could find them. She never mentioned pain or adversity. But she inspired a generation with her determination and grace.

My mother had rheumatoid arthritis that started before I was born and led her to spend the last thirty years of her life in a wheelchair. She

---

[56] John Bright-Fey, *A Morning Cup of Tai Chi* (China: Crane Hill Publishing, Inc. 2006).

created beauty everywhere she went and blessed the lives of her family and friends, even as she struggled with increasing deformity and her world became smaller and smaller. She was often in pain, but she never complained. Even after she had small strokes and could not manage life on her own, her courage and resourcefulness was a model for handling tough times. I was grateful for her spirit staying strong and interested in every detail, even when her life became so limited. With such examples, I was blessed.

Looking back, I realize that the wonder of being human is our capacity to grow and to use adversity to be stronger and better. Through tragedy and illness, more than any other events in our lives, we hone resilience, find inner strength, and enhance our abilities to understand one another. Even depression may confer the benefit of seeing reality more clearly! Fortunately, there is built into us all a potential to rise above our circumstances and seek noble solutions. Doing that may be easier if we have a mentor or a healing presence, but even the most deprived person can find the way on his or her own and be an inspiration to others. I hope this book helps you with your quest along the way.

APPENDIX A:

UNCONSCIOUS DEFENSE MECHANISMS:

The Grant Study divided defense mechanisms into mature, anxious or neurotic, immature, and psychotic defenses. These are all unconscious or semi-conscious responses to anxiety that affect everyone even the healthiest of people. Everyone has some mature defenses, some immature defenses and lots of anxious defenses. We cannot escape them and they all distort reality to some extent.

Mature Defenses

So-called mature defenses are also known as *coping mechanisms*. They result in activities such as helping others, engaging in humor or artistic expression, or getting on with the business of the day. The great thing about mature defenses is that they tend to bind us to others, giving us added support in anxious times.

A friend, Florence Sawyer, was a successful businesswoman and a happily married mother of three when she discovered a lump in her breast. The doctor recommended a mastectomy. Florence had many friends, and they all flocked to her side to see what they could do. When I walked into her room three days after the surgery, she was smiling and invited me to sit down. I felt very emotional and sad that her hard work and success had been interrupted by this threat to her life. Florence saw my distress and rushed to reassure me. "It's not so bad," she said. "I've been trying to lose five pounds for the longest time, and they made it easy for me!" Her humor helped me get over being so emotional, and we were able to talk about her situation.

Clearly, her humor helped her through the tough time and also bound her friends to her.

Mature defenses help us cope. These are the skills that see us through difficulty and are good ones to emulate. Mature defenses should be encouraged wherever they occur.

Neurotic (Anxious) Defenses

Neurotic (or, in other words, anxious) defenses block anxiety and often lead to symptoms that prompt people to see a doctor or psychiatrist, where they may get the care and support they need for underlying emotional issues. These defenses include hysteria or pseudo-neurological symptoms, phobias, obsessive-compulsive symptoms, rationalizations, intellectualization and reaction formation.

Ruby Mae Roland was admitted to the hospital with a pseudo-paralysis. After we talked for a while, I told her that her symptom was a sign of anxiety. "I can't imagine why I would be anxious now," she said, looking puzzled. "I've been through chemotherapy twice, all on my own. I took care of myself even when I was sick with pneumonia last winter. I've been doing well. The doctor says this new pain isn't cancer—it's a strained muscle. Besides, I'm a strong person. What is going on? Why now?" She looked at me, hoping for an answer.

"Tell me what was going on in your life just before these symptoms started," I replied, trying to get more information to understand her situation.

She looked away from me, trying to remember. She smiled slightly, and a look of deep sorrow crept into her eyes. After a minute she said, "My favorite niece was killed in a shooting in Chicago this summer. She had agreed to take care of me at the end, when I couldn't take care of myself anymore. It gave me great peace to think I wouldn't be alone in my time of trouble." She had identified the source of her anxiety. As we talked some more, I could see that she had already begun the process of thinking through what she would do next.

Neurotic or anxious defenses, like pseudo-paralysis, are either benign (like rationalizations) or serious enough to take an individual to the doctor for needed help and support. Treatment is aimed at clarifying what the anxiety is all about and helping the patient find a way out. Those who also have depression probably engage immature defenses (self-defeating behaviors) as well. This is not a conscious choice, but is the best that person can do at the moment to protect against being overwhelmed.

Immature Defenses

Immature defenses are behaviors or reactions we associate with the young and with people who we say have *personality disorders.* We also see immature defenses in people who are faced with chronic illness or those who lead difficult lives. They are also present in depression.

Immature defenses give rise to self-defeating behavior that must be addressed if the patient is to do better. Immature defenses protect an individual from anxiety, but they tend to alienate others (or at least create distance); this removes support and encouragement at a time when they might be helpful.

Immature defenses include somatization (physical symptoms, especially pain, brought on by stress), hypochondriasis (preoccupation with being ill in spite of medical evidence to the contrary), paranoia (denial of one's own impulses that are then ascribed to others, either groups or individuals), passive-aggressive behavior (such as being uncooperative, being late, leaving messes, or forgetting things), fantasy (such as imagining success to avoid facing failure, or claiming noble motives to disguise ignoble behavior), and so-called "acting-out" behavior, such as doing something unwise or being impulsive without thinking through consequences.

Joyce Cole was a recovering alcoholic who had sustained severe injuries in a car wreck. She was sent to see me because she still had lot of pain after a year and was also dealing with depression. She was an angry woman who resisted most suggestions that might benefit her. I did eventually convince her to come to group therapy to work out her considerable distress over her children. As she came to group the first day, I noticed she had new bandages on her arm.

"I'm so afraid my son is going to get killed," she reported to the group when her turn came to introduce herself and talk about her problems. "He came home from Chicago after a man threatened to kill him. Now he wants to go back and fight the man. I've been pleading with him not to go." Members of the group agreed that he should not go.

"What happened to you?" I asked, pointing to the bandage on her arm.

"I got into a fight with my neighbor. She always plays her TV too loud and got right in my face when I told her to turn it down. I was sick of her lip, so I let her have it." Here she was, having difficulty recovering from previous injuries, and she got into a physical fight? Her impulsive, self-defeating behavior was a good example of an immature defense.

I appealed to the group. "What do the rest of you think about solving problems this way?" I could always depend on the wisdom of the group to confront self-defeating behavior. "Maybe you can use this as an example to your son of how not to handle problems with others," I added. "You may feel better, but you can get hurt, or worse—and it doesn't solve anything!"

Studies show that the immature defenses of hypochondriasis and somatization are common in those with chronic pain and in those who are chronically ill or threatened with medical illness. These symptoms are also common with depression, schizophrenia, and in lonely, frightened people. Patients using immature defenses need to be seen more often so that they stay well and do not have to be in pain or sick to get in to the doctor.

Immature defenses provide immediate relief and are common in children dealing with anxiety. What parent doesn't know the stomach ache or the fantastic story when a child is under stress? Immature defenses are also used by people who are overwhelmed with complicated life situations. But even the healthiest among us use immature defenses from time to time.

Psychotic and Narcissistic Defenses

Finally, psychotic or narcissistic defenses are those we see in mental illness or severe medical illness, or when there is a mental breakdown from extreme stress or mental confusion from a medical cause or dementia. Although all defense mechanisms distort reality somewhat, psychosis is being out of touch with it; it can include delusions and hallucination. Delusions are false beliefs that are not culturally consistent: they would not seem real to any sane person. Hallucinations are sensory experiences that are generated by the individual.

Joe Taylor was a patient who suffered from a psychosis. Joe had severe kidney disease and was admitted to the hospital for dialysis. One day, I got an emergency call: Joe had stabbed the man in the next bed with a syringe. Joe was restrained in bed when I got to the ward, and the police were hovering nearby.

"That man's trying to kill me!" Joe said when I asked him what had happened. "People keep tying me down, sticking me, putting something in my nose." Even though he was correct about those things, he was obviously confused and disoriented. He did not know the time of day, or where or why he was in the hospital. This delirium had been brought on by chemical changes in his blood from the dialysis and other medical problems. The police left after I was able to explain to them that Joe had become confused and had reacted out of feeling threatened. We moved Joe to a well-lit private room and had his family sit with him to keep him oriented while the doctors addressed his electrolyte balance.

APPENDIX B

MEDICAL CONDITIONS THAT MAY GIVE RISE TO DEPRESSION:

Neurological:
Epilepsy
Stroke10-27%
Multiple sclerosis: 40%
Parkinson's disease: 40%
Huntington's chorea
Dementia
Trauma to the brain

Cardiovascular:
Heart attack: 40–65%
Coronary heart disease: 18–20%

Endocrine:
Hypothyroidism
Hyperthyroidism
Hypoparathyroidism
Hyperparathyroidism

Cancer(especially lung and pancreas): 25%

Infectious:
    Syphilis
    Lyme disease
    AIDS

Metabolic:
    Diabetes 25%
    Porphyria
    Wilson's disease
    Pellagra (vitamin B3 deficiency)

Other: After surgery
    Neuroendocrine dysautonomia

APPENDIX C

MEDICATIONS THAT MAY CAUSE DEPRES-
SION ESPECIALLY IN THE ELDERLY

Accutane: Treats acne.
Alcohol
Antabuse: Treats alcoholism.
Anticonvulsants: Epilepsy -examples Celontin and Zarontin.
Barbiturates: phenobarbital and secobarbital.
Benzodiazepines: Ativan, Dalmane, Halcion, Klonopin, Librium, Va-
lium, and Xanax.
Beta-adrenergic blockers: Lopressor, Tenormin and Coreg.
Bromocriptine (Parlodel): Treats Parkinson's disease.
Calcium-channel blockers: Calan, Cardizem, Tiazac, and Procardia.
Estrogens: Premarin and Prempro.
Fluoroquinolone antibiotics: Cipro and Floxin.
Interferon alfa: Treats cancers, hepatitis B and C.
Norplant: birth control.
Opioids: codeine, morphine, Demerol, Percodan, and OxyContin.
Statins: Mevacor, Zocor, Pravachol, Lescol, and Lipitor.
Zovirax: Treats shingles and herpes

APPENDIX D

SYMPTOMS OF DEPRESSION

According to the National Institute of Mental Health, symptoms of depression may include the following:

Difficulty concentrating, remembering details, and making decisions

Fatigue and decreased energy

Feelings of guilt, worthlessness, and/or helplessness

Feelings of hopelessness and/or pessimism

Insomnia, early-morning wakefulness, or excessive sleeping

Irritability, restlessness

Loss of interest in activities or hobbies once pleasurable, including sex

Overeating or appetite loss

Persistent aches or pains, headaches, cramps, or digestive problems that do not ease even with treatment

Persistent sad, anxious, or *empty* feelings

Thoughts of suicide, suicide attempts

APPENDIX E

PLAN FOR TREATING BAD PAIN PERIODS

Just as we need routines for exercise and breathing, everyone needs to have a plan for managing bad pain periods—times when they do too much or when the weather is bad, or when they are under increased stress. This is important, because it is too easy to get discouraged and depressed when pain returns again and again. And it is also too easy to get lazy and stop exercising. So have a plan. Recognizing these pitfalls is part of managing your life.

An effective plan will lessen disruption to your life. First, know which events might increase your pain. You might even keep a diary to track various triggers: the weather, certain foods, too much sitting, or failure to exercise and stretch. Then, include all the activities below in your plan:

- Get more rest, but not for more than three to four days
- Increase the dose of medication for a few days
- Or change to another medicine
- Drink more water
- Do some stretching and movement
- Use meditation
- Engage in an interesting hobby that distracts from the pain
- Use heat or ice
- Use light therapy or a transcutaneous electrical nerve stimulation (TENS) unit

Opiates and other pain medication must be only a part of your pain management package.

As the pain gets better, have a plan to get going again. This plan includes getting up, getting dressed, having a stretching and moving routine, participating in useful activities and occupations, and being with other people. Enjoy your recovery!

For specific activities you can do for yourself, read: *Heal Thyself! What You Can Do To Recover From Chronic Pain and Depression* by Dr. Carmichael coming out soon.

Made in the USA
San Bernardino, CA
22 December 2013